BE STAY FIT!

Why Your Workout Doesn't Work... And How to Fix It

Sgt. Davis & Troop 9,
all the best!
Dr. Paul

Dr. Paul Kennedy
Foreword by Matt Brzycki

Blue River Press
Indianapolis, Indiana

LCCN: 2002114950

Cover designed by Phil Velikan
Cover photography by Stockbyte, www.stockbyte.com
Interior photography by Paul Kennedy

Printed in the United States of America
10 9 8 7 6 5 4 3 2 1

Distributed in the United States by
Cardinal Publishers Group
7301 Georgetown Road, Suite 118
Indianapolis, Indiana 46268
www.cardinalpub.com

This book is dedicated to my father, Major Paul E. Kennedy, who died in the service of his country when I was too young to know him. His memory and his courage against long odds have served as a constant inspiration to me throughout my lifetime.

And to the memory of my mother, his widow Leota, whose own quiet courage helped sustain me and teach me the true meaning of ethics and the importance of doing the right thing, I humbly dedicate this book.

— Paul M. Kennedy, Ed. D.
October 2002

Table of Contents

Many fitness and weight management programs fail because they lack one of the three major components of a comprehensive training program. This chapter will explore those major components and suggest ways to combine them into a total fitness and weight management package that will produce results on a regular basis.

For most people, fitness programs are a situation of too much too soon. Understanding how to set meaningful and measurable goals can be the difference between fitness program failure and long-term success. This chapter will provide information on how to set realistic yet achievable goals that will keep you motivated. In addition, processing feedback and results from each training session will help to keep you on track throughout your program.

Intensity is the real key to success in any fitness program whether the exercise is of an aerobic or anaerobic nature. This chapter will focus on ways of increasing and/or improving intensity and, thereby, improve results. Focus will be placed on proper technique, especially as it pertains to strength training, and more efficient training methodologies.

Chapter Four: 57
Diet is a Four-Letter Word

Diets are NOT the way to approach weight management and/or weight loss. Eating plans, on the other hand, can represent a permanent and realistic approach to food as a means to a long-term lifestyle change that can survive in the real world in which we live. A basic understanding of the role food plays as well as measuring REAL food consumption can go far toward creating a successful and lifelong relationship with the food that we eat. The Food Pyramid becomes the backdrop for nutritional success.

Chapter Five: 71
Understanding Body Composition

Body composition changes and not just "weight loss" are the real goals of a fitness program that will produce permanent results. Fundamental information about assessing your body's composition will be presented and discussed. Additionally, the contribution of lean body mass to PERMANENT fat loss will be demonstrated and explained.

Chapter Six: 83
Getting Started: Putting it All Together

Two of the most challenging aspects to a fitness program are getting started and, then, putting all the elements together. Simple and fundamentally sound starter programs known as "Core Programs" will be outlined and discussed. Further, a point system for combining all of the elements of a total fitness program will be presented to leave the reader, whether a novice or experienced exerciser, with a "real world" fitness program that they can understand and use.

Author's Note

Each chapter of *Be Fit, Stay Fit!*, with the exception of the final chapter, will be followed by answers to real fitness questions collected by the author over the years. These "real world questions" will provide a support mechanism to the basic content of each chapter and will reinforce each chapter's theme. The reader will probably recognize many of the questions as ones that they would like to have asked or have always wanted to ask. This format will add a "real world" flavor to the content and will allow the reader to relate to each chapter in a more personal way.

Due to content complexity, some chapters are somewhat more involved than others since some total fitness concepts require greater explanation and concomitant treatment. All content will be readable, entertaining and easy to understand. With this understanding is empowerment!

Paul M. Kennedy, Ed.D.
October 2002

Foreword

It is quite an honor to be chosen to pen the introduction to the first of what I hope to be many books by Dr. Paul Kennedy. I have had the pleasure of knowing Dr. Kennedy since the early 1980s when he was a graduate student at Penn State and advisor to the Penn State Barbell Club. As an undergraduate student, I had the distinct privilege of doing an internship in strength and conditioning with him in the fall of 1982.

In the early part 1984, Dr. Kennedy was named the Strength and Conditioning Coach at Rutgers University. In August of that year, he hired me as the Assistant Strength and Conditioning Coach and I worked for him in that capacity until July 1990.

As my supervisor, Dr. Kennedy was the consummate mentor and role model. His professional image has been a never-ending inspiration to me. He was — and continues to be — an endless source of valuable information and infinite wisdom. I can honestly say that hardly a day went by where I did not learn something from Dr. Kennedy.

I feel extremely fortunate to have been groomed by an individual such as Dr. Kennedy. Much of what I have been able to accomplish in the fitness industry is a direct result of his mentoring. Dr. Kennedy has had a profound impact on my development as a strength and fitness professional. And I am proud to say that I have patterned much of my style after him.

Dr. Kennedy is a dynamic, informative, articulate and riveting speaker — and you will find that his writing is the same. In an industry that, unfortunately, is overflowing with underhanded, unscrupulous and unsavory entrepreneurs as well as a multitude of self-proclaimed "experts" and "authorities," Dr. Kennedy is a man of honesty, loyalty and integrity. Having been employed as a strength and fitness professional at the collegiate level since 1983, it is my opinion that Dr. Kennedy is one of the most credible sources of information on strength and fitness in the world.

Let Dr. Kennedy and his first book be your guide to be fit and staying fit.

Matt Brzycki
Coordinator of Recreational
Fitness and Wellness Programs
Princeton University
September 26, 2002

Chapter One
The Major Components of Fitness — An Overview

Most fitness programs fail because they are one dimensional or too narrowly focused. The fact of the matter is that fitness has many components and all need to be addressed if the fitness program is to be successful. It is not unusual, for example, to observe a fitness center or recreational facility where most of the males are strength training in a haphazard and disorganized manner in the "weight room" and most of the females are doing aerobic activities at less than optimal or even challenging levels in the cardiovascular center. Both are making a mistake. Although adequate and/or optimal exercise intensity will be addressed in Chapter Three, it should be obvious that any individual who concentrates on only one aspect of the fitness spectrum is not optimizing their results and may actually be doing more harm than good. That's because all of the components of fitness are important and, in many ways, interdependent.

The major components of fitness are: cardiorespiratory (more commonly known as cardiovascular or "cardio") fitness, muscular strength and endurance, flexibility and body composition. The relationship between all of these components will become apparent as you read this book. However, combining them into an effective, safe and time-efficient program is the true purpose of the pages that follow. Additionally, learning and understanding how much execise is sufficient to improve general fitness will be an underlying theme. Since most individuals either undertrain (do too little) or overtrain (do too much), finding the right amount of exercise can be confusing and is the main reason why most workout programs fail. Once you understand how much exercise you need and how to measure it in a simple and concise manner, the guess work is minimized and staying motivated for the long-term becomes easier simply due to the fact that you now know where you're going and where you've been in terms of your fitness levels. And what's more, it's easy to do and simple to track! But let's first take a look at the components individually.

CARDIORESPIRATORY FITNESS

Oxygen equals energy and the more oxygen that the body can breathe in and deliver to the cells, the more energy can be produced to accomplish a task. It doesn't matter if the task is lifting some weights, running a few miles or carrying the groceries from the store to the car. If the body can't get enough oxygen it responds by increasing its heart rate as well as the rate of breathing. That's because the circulatory system (the heart and blood vessels) "picks up" the oxygen in the lungs and delivers it to the working muscles of the body. The more efficiently that these systems exchange oxygen and deliver it throughout the body, the more energy we seem to have and the more work we can perform without being fatigued or "winded".

The cardiorespiratory or cardiovascular system responds dramatically to the old adage, "If you don't use it, you'll lose it." In other words, inactivity—especially for extended periods of time—causes these interconnected systems to lose efficiency over time and causes us to become less fit. Human beings were created to move on a regular basis and recent evidence has suggested that this basic principle is even in our genetic code! So when we stop moving or exercising on a regular basis, we actually start to allow ourselves to become diseased and, perhaps, commit a slow form of physiological suicide by causing our cardiorespiratory and cardiovascular systems to deteriorate. But the good news is that the dramatic response that our body has to *inactivity* is mirrored by the dramatic response that it has to any form of activity that moderately or even minimally challenges the heart, lungs and circulatory system.

What this means is that any individual can improve their level of "cardio" fitness and that the exercise—or challenge—does *not* have to be prolonged or harsh to have an effect. In fact, it is becoming more and more clear that doing moderate forms of cardiovascular exercise on a regular basis over time is a safer and more effective way to train the body to improve gradually and progressively. The idea, of course, is to challenge the body to do just slightly more than it is used to doing in order to elicit what is known as a "training effect." How much is enough? It is recommended that cardiovascular training take place at least three to five days per week with three days being sufficient for someone just starting out on a program. It is also recommended that the time frame for such training be a minimum of 20 to 30 minutes. However, it should be noted that recent evidence is beginning to suggest that almost any type of cardiovascular activity (such as walking, running, biking, swimming or even mowing the lawn—push mowers only, please) that is done in bouts of 10 minutes or so throughout the day and totaling 20 to 30 minutes (or more) can be nearly as effective in improving cardiovascular fitness levels as doing the exercise in an uninterrupted time frame of 20 to 30 minutes.

Engaging in activities that challenge the heart, lungs and circulatory system (also known as "aerobic exercise") on a regular and progressive basis will improve the body's ability to:

1. Pump more blood per beat (known as stroke volume)
2. Carry more blood to the cells
3. Increase capillary density (the areas of the body where oxygen is exchanged from the lungs to the blood and from the blood to the cells)
4. Improve the elasticity of the arteries and veins which helps to promote blood flow
5. Increase the strength of the cardiac muscle (known as the heart)
6. Breathe in more air (and, therefore, more oxygen) due to an increase in the strength of the diaphragm
7. Help reduce the incidence or growth of arterial plaque (the fatty substance that can clog arteries and significantly reduce or block blood flow)
8. Strengthen the skeletal system
9. Lower blood pressure
10. Regulate insulin uptake (which is of particular concern to those with non-insulin dependent diabetes).

As you can see, these improvements will allow the body to perform any task more efficiently and effectively and positively effect general health.

Get FITT!

Cardiovascular training adheres to a principle known as the FITT Principle. This is simply an acronym for the four fundamental components of a cardiovascular program. The first component (F) stands for frequency. Discussed earlier, it is recommended that cardiovascular training take place three to five days per week. The second component (I) stands for intensity. This means that the heart rate must reach a level that will produce what is known as a "training effect." The formula for determining the suggested levels necessary to produce the training effect is presented in Chapter Three. The third component (T) stands for time—the amount of time necessary to engage in a specific activity to produce a training effect . This time frame is generally considered to be a minimum of 20 to 30 minutes to a maximum of approximately one hour. For beginners, it may be necessary to start with even shorter time frames and intensities and these will also be discussed and presented in Chapter Three. The last component (T) stands for type or the kind of activity to be completed. Any exercise that is rhythmic in nature and involves large muscle groups can be defined as an aerobic exercise. Examples of cardiovascular or aerobic exercise are brisk walking, running, biking, rowing and swimming but even hiking and working in the garden can be considered in this category if they are sufficiently intense and result in an increased heart rate due to the activity.

Therefore, cardiovascular training should be a regular and integral part of any fitness program. Improved endurance through training will enhance one's ability to increase muscular strength and can have an impact on improvements in body composition. More information on setting up and implementing a cardiovascular program will be presented in Chapter Three.

MUSCULAR STRENGTH AND MUSCULAR ENDURANCE

Muscular strength is defined as the ability to complete a single repetition with a maximum amount of resistance or weight. Muscular endurance, on the other hand, is the ability to complete many repetitions with a *sub*maximum amount of resistance or weight. What this means is that any exercise or activity that can be completed for more than one repetition must be considered and measured as muscular endurance. Clearly, there is a relationship between the ability to lift or move a maximum resistance or weight for just one repetition and the ability to lift a lighter weight or resistance for multiple repetitions. However, training to improve muscular strength need not—and probably should not— be accomplished using single repetitions. Optimal repetition ranges for the vast majority of individuals for gaining strength appears to be about 8 to 12 repetitions for the upper body musculature and about 10 to 15 repetitions for the lower body musculature. Moreover, unless one is engaged in competitive weightlifting (as opposed to strength training or strength fitness), attempting single repetitions with maximum resistance is unnecessary and, in some case, may cause injury.

Most individuals mistakenly feel that the weight room or strength training facility is a place to demonstrate their strength rather than improve it. The result is set after set of relatively meaningless low-repetition exercise that may not stimulate the muscle tissue optimally. Indeed, it has been suggested that the most important factor in training to gain strength is the amount of time spent in uninterrupted contraction time and that the optimal time frame for that uninterrupted contraction is about 35 to 75 seconds. Therefore, most low-repetition sets of exercise that emphasize only the concentric phase of the lift (the phase in which the weight or resistance is raised) and de-emphasize the eccentric phase of the lift (the phase in which the weight or resistance is lowered under control) do not allow the muscle(s) to remain in contraction time long enough to optimize results.

With the information on proper exercise form presented in Chapter Three, it will be easy to see that this optimal time frame suggested above is easily and safely achieved with each set of exercise or with each lift since the resistance is taught to be lifted, moved or raised and lowered in a controlled manner. Each repetition, therefore, is accomplished in approximately three to six seconds and is completed through a full range of motion. (Proper strength training form and technique will be described and presented in Chapter Three). In this way, both muscular strength and muscular endurance can be achieved safely and efficiently.

The cornerstone theory surrounding the ability of the body to gain strength is known as "Progressive Resistance." This means that each time a muscle or group of muscles is trained, it must be coaxed into doing slightly more muscular work than it accomplished previously. The body responds to this additional workload by retaining more proteins in the form of amino acids and, if given a sufficient time to recover from the new and increased challenge (which we call a "workout"), it will improve slightly in strength and, possibly, size. Size gains and, to a lesser degree, strength gains are largely genetically determined and, therefore, comparing oneself to others that may be more genetically "gifted" can sometimes be a frustrating and demotivating experience. But EVERY individual has the ability to improve the strength and endurance of their musculoskeletal system by training it carefully and progressively.

The human musculoskeletal system is really nothing more than a system of levers. Each muscle is attached to one or more bones (the levers) and when the muscles contract or are trained to contract, the bones to which they are attached move. This is how human movement or locomotion is achieved. The tissue that attaches the muscles to the bones is known as a tendon. It is this tissue that, many times, becomes sore if the muscle is asked to do significantly more work than it is used to doing. As one can infer, stronger muscles with greater endurance can improve the efficiency of every movement and task and, thereby, allow an individual to act and feel more fit—because they are!

It is also important to understand that every individual has different potentials and limitations when it comes to muscular strength and endurance. The factors regarding those potentials and limitations will be briefly discussed in the next chapter on goal setting. But understand that the best person to compare yourself to in terms of results and fitness program improvements is yourself. Any other comparisons are essentially meaningless due to the many different genetic factors that control the final outcome of any fitness program.

FLEXIBILITY

Flexibility is defined as the ability to move through an optimal range of motion. This is particularly true of the major joints of the body and, therefore, flexibility is many times described as joint range of motion. By improving joint range of motion, movements are accomplished more easily and, since the muscles surrounding the joint can move more freely, power is enhanced. Many people feel that resistance training will cause the body to "bulk up" and become less flexible and, therefore, they avoid strength training as a regular part of their comprehensive fitness program. This is a major mistake since, indeed, it is possible to improve both strength and flexibility at the same time. Again, proper form and technique is the key. Additionally, many people spend little time stretching the muscles and connective tissue in terms of "holding" the stretching movement.

There are two basic types of stretching that are known as "active" and "passive" stretching. Active stretching, which has a tendency to effect the softer tissues of the muscles rather than the somewhat more dense connective tissues, can be accomplished by engaging in activities that simulate the movement or movements that are be involved in a chosen activity. Swinging a golf club a few times before actually striking the ball or performing light agility drills before engaging in a basketball game would be good examples of active stretching. Clearly, caution must be taken with this type of stretching technique to be sure that the muscles and connective tissues are properly and gradually "warmed-up" before engaging in movements that, due to their speed, may overchallenge the joints and cause injury.

With passive stretching, more of the elongating effect of the movement is transferred to the connective tissues such as the tendons (the tissues that connect the muscle to the bone) and the stretching movement is maintained in what is known as a "static" position. This means that a specific "stretch" is held in a fixed position for a specific period of time (usually about 15 to 30 seconds). Passive stretching also involves achieving a stretch position that is challenging — in other words a slight tug is felt during the stretch—that helps to increase the existing range of motion. The stretching movement should be taken only to the point of a mild discomfort and never to the point of pain. In this way, the range of motion can be gradually increased over time. "Static" stretching (described in more detail below) is a typical passive stretch technique.

Stretching Technique

Stretching technique is a critical factor in successfully preparing the muscles and connective tissue for activity. There are two types of stretching techniques. The first is known as "ballistic" stretching and involves rapid and, possibly, uncontrolled bouncing movements. This technique, because of its speed of movement, can and will produce high force over a brief time frame and, therefore, may expose the joint and soft tissue to injury. It has been suggested that this type of flexibility movement has a place in preparing for certain sport-specific movements which, theoretically, prepares the joints and soft tissues for "explosive" movements. However, the effectiveness of this technique—as well as its safety compared to the effectiveness of the slower and more controlled technique called "static" stretching—is somewhat questionable.

Static stretching (a passive stretching technique) involves a slow, controlled and prolonged "holding" of the stretch position through a complete and full range of motion. The stretch position is held for approximately 15 to 30 seconds at a point that produces a "tugging" on the muscle and connective tissue. It is not unusual for the stretch position, therefore, to elicit a mild level of discomfort. By slowly moving into the stretch position, holding the stretch for the specified time frame suggested above and subsequently "releasing" the stretch slowly, the range of motion of the muscles and connective tissues can be easily and safely enhanced.

Many flexibility routines or programs fail not only due to improper or unsafe technique, but also because they are performed with "cold" muscles. It is always a good idea to engage in a slow and/or gradual warm-up of the body before beginning any stretching program. By slightly increasing the body's "core" temperature and by increasing blood flow to the muscles with activities such as light calisthenics or exercising on a stationary bike for a period of about 5 or 10 minutes, the body is better prepared to accept and respond to the adjustments created by either passive or active stretching techniques. Additionally, it is important to involve both active and passive techniques in a comprehensive flexibility program that will enhance not only range of motion, but will, as a result, improve performance in any chosen activity.

Another reason why flexibility programs fail is a lack of frequency. It is important to stretch daily and not just when one is about to participate in an activity. After all, life is an activity and improved range of motion can allow anyone to participate in it with greater ease of movement and, perhaps, less pain and injury. There is no doubt that stretching on a regular basis is superior to stretching "every once in a while" and that range of motion is improved with a regular schedule of stretching when compared to stretching maybe once or twice per week. While there is some controversy concerning whether stretching should take place before or after an activity, a gentle and controlled "active" type of stretching would appear to be helpful before an activity while "passive" stretching techniques would be helpful for specific problem areas, such as the lower back and hamstrings, both before and after an activity. Stretching immediately following a specific strength training exercise or cardiovascular activity, therefore, would be considered an optimal way of increasing the flexibility of areas of the body that are somewhat "tight" or less flexible than others.

It should also be noted that as we age, and particularly if we have been inactive, we have a tendency to become less flexible. The reasons have to do with a lack of retained moisture in the connective tissue itself—in other words the body is "drying up" a little bit—and, probably more importantly, a slight enlargement of the fibers that make up these same connective tissues that surround and protect the joint. For this reason, flexibility training becomes an even more crucial part of every fitness training program after we reach the age of about 25 or 30.

Some simple passive stretching exercises for several of the more common "problem areas" are demonstrated on the following pages. Remember that the stretching position should be held for about 15 to 30 seconds, or more if desired or deemed appropriate, and that the flexibility training should be accomplished after a sufficient warm-up. Assume the stretch position slowly and carefully. After the position has been held for the desired time frame, slowly return to the original position. If problem areas exist, it is also a good idea to stretch those areas immediately before and after strength training them. And speaking of exercising, there is no better way to *enhance* flexibility than by strength training the muscle or joint through a *full range of motion* (more on that in Chapter Three).

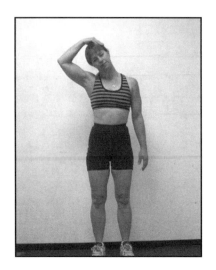 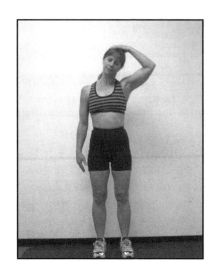

Lateral Neck Stretch

Stand with your feet approximately shoulder width apart and with an erect posture. Tilt the head to the left side until a stretch is felt on the side of the neck on the opposite side. As illustrated, it is possible to gently assist with the stretch by placing the left hand on the right side of the head. Hold the stretch for 15 to 30 seconds. Return to the neutral position and repeat on the opposite side.

Standing Pectoral and Anterior Deltoid Stretch

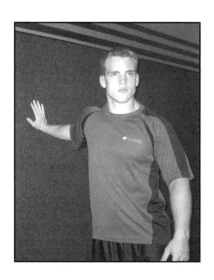

Stand perpendicular to and approximately at arms length away from the wall. As illustrated, place the hand closest to the wall on the wall at the same level as the shoulder joint. Gently lean with the torso forward and slightly away from the wall while maintaining hand contact with the wall. Hold the stretch for 15 to 30 seconds. Return to a neutral position and repeat on the opposite side.

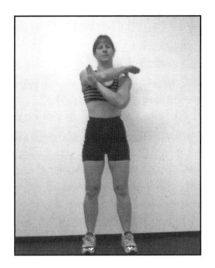
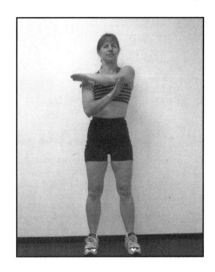

Posterior Deltoid Stretch

Stand with feet shoulder-width apart. As illustrated, bend the left arm at the elbow, raise to shoulder level in front of the body with palm down. Place the right hand behind the elbow and gently pull across the midline of the body. Hold the stretch for 15 to 30 seconds. Return to a neutral position and repeat on the opposite side.

Low Back Stretch

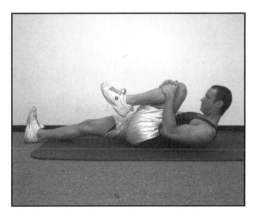

Lie supine (face up) preferably on a padded surface or a mat. As illustrated, raise the left knee to the chest while allowing the right leg to remain straight and in contact with the floor. Place the hands just below the left knee and gently pull in toward the chest while raising the head off the mat or floor. Hold the stretch for 15 to 30 seconds. Return to the neutral position and repeat on the opposite side.

Standing Hamstring Stretch

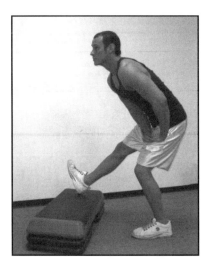

Stand facing a low bench or slightly raised surface. As illustrated, extend the right leg and place the heel of the right leg on the bench or raised surface. Place left and right hand on the thigh of the slightly bent left leg. Slowly lower the hips while leaning slightly forward and keeping the right leg straight to establish the stretch position for the right hamstring. Hold the stretch for 15 to 30 seconds. Return to the neutral position and repeat on the opposite side.

Seated Hamstring, Low Back and Hip Stretch

Sit on a padded surface or mat. As illustrated, place the sole of the right foot against the inner thigh of the extended left leg.

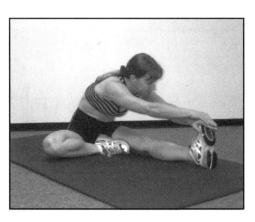

The toes of the left foot should remain pointed towards the ceiling. Place the right hand over the left hand and slowly lean forward. Attempt to touch the toes of the left foot. Continue to lean forward until a gentle tug is felt in either the left hamstring or lower back. Hold the stretch at this point for 15 to 30 seconds. *Do not over extend.* Return to the neutral position and repeat on the opposite side. This flexibility exercise is not recommended for those individuals with recurrent knee or lower back pain.

Quadricep (Thigh) Stretch

Stand facing the back of a chair or other similarly stationary object. As illustrated, place the right hand on the back of the chair for stabilization. Bring the heel up toward the hip by bending the left leg. Grasp the left ankle with the left hand and continue to draw the heel toward the hip until a stretch is felt on the front of the left thigh. Hold for 15 to 30 seconds. Return to the neutral position and repeat on the opposite side.

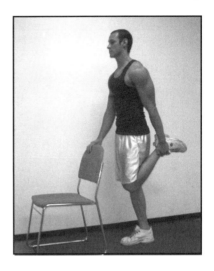

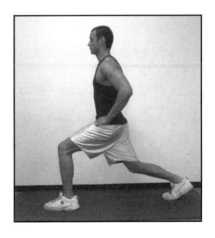

Inner Thigh and Groin Stretch

As illustrated, place the bottom of the feet together and draw the heels toward the hip. As shown, position the hands on the ankles and place the elbows against the inside of each thigh. Gently push down with the elbows against the thigh until a stretch is felt on the inner thigh. Hold the stretch for 15 to 30 seconds.

Hip Flexor Stretch

From a standing position with the hands on the hips, step forward to a somewhat elongated stride position, as shown. Slowly lower the hips vertically until a stretch is felt in the groin area. Hold the stretch for 15 to 30 seconds. Carefully return to the neutral position by stepping forward and repeat on the opposite side.

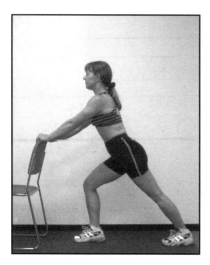

Gastrocnemius (Calf) Stretch

Stand facing the back of a chair or other similarly stationary object. As illustrated, place both hands on the back of the chair or stable object. Step back with the left leg to a position where a stretch is felt just above the back of the heel. Lean slightly forward while keeping the bottom of the foot, including the heel, flat to the mat or floor surface. Hold the stretch for 15 to 30 seconds. Slowly step forward to the neutral position and repeat on the opposite side.

These ten simple flexibility exercises can and should be repeated as deemed appropriate and necessary before, during and after any general exercise routine or program. Indeed, stretching immediately following a workout or exercise routine can help to reduce recovery time and can decrease or prevent what is commonly known as "delayed-onset muscle soreness."

Flexibility Assessment

Now we are going to look at a very simple assessment of overall flexibility called *The Sit and Reach Test*. It is simple to set

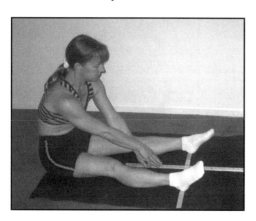

up and even more simple to complete and to score. All that is needed is a flat surface to sit on, a yardstick or a cloth measuring tape and some one-inch cloth adhesive tape. As shown in the photo, sit on the floor with the feet about 12 inches apart. Place the yardstick or measuring tape midway between the heels with the zero mark closest to the body. The heels should be aligned on the piece of cloth adhesive tape at the 15-inch mark on the yardstick or measuring tape. Place one hand on top of the other, as shown, with the tips of the fingers aligned and gently lean forward

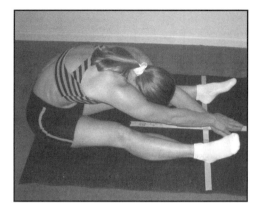

while exhaling and dropping the head between the arms. Maintain contact with the yardstick or measuring tape while keeping the knees straight. The score is the farthest point reached measured in inches from the zero point, after three tries. Establish your base level (current flexibility level) and record your score periodically (about every two or three weeks) at the space provided at the bottom of your *Body Composition Measurements* card in Appendix C. This will help to show your progress as you become more flexible!

Body Composition

Most individuals (nearly 85%) begin a fitness program with the idea of losing weight. Generally, however, most of these same individuals don't realize that some of the weight, in some cases most of the weight, that they lose is either water or protein. What they really want to lose is fat and this is where understanding body *composition* and not just body *weight* is so important. A more specific look at body composition will be presented in Chapter Five. However, understanding that body weight is more than just a number on a scale is the first step toward realizing the reasons why most "weight management" programs fail over and over again.

Simply, the body's weight is composed of two types of tissue or "mass." The first type of mass is known as "fat-free" mass or lean-body mass (LBM) and consists of muscles, bone and other internal organs. The rest is know as "adipose tissue" or fat. Even the blood contains some amount, hopefully a small amount , of fat. The idea, in most cases, is to reduce the amount of fat and increase the amount of fat-free mass. So it is body *composition* and not just body *weight* that must be measured and modified to reach a specific and healthier level. Metabolism (the rate at which we burn calories), is largely determined by the amount of fat-free mass and plays a large role in the success of a weight management and fitness program. But more on that in Chapter Five. At this point, it is important to know that most weight management programs fail in the long-term because of a singular reliance on scale weight. As you will see later in the book, there is a better and more permanent way to lose the fat and be more fit.

FREQUENTLY ASKED QUESTIONS

I do lots of sit-ups and bench presses but I still can't seem to lose much weight and I still have a "gut." What am I doing wrong?

Although you have increased the strength of your abdomen and chest, you have done little to help your body burn more calories for two reasons. First, you are training only two major muscle groups which will do little to increase your metabolic rate (the rate at which you burn calories) because you are excluding most of the other major muscle groups, particularly those of the lower body. This means that the lean-body tissue that will help to promote or increase your metabolism is not being trained optimally. For example, by including strength training exercises for your upper back, shoulders, hips and legs in addition to your current program, you will increase muscle mass or lean-body tissue all over your body instead of just the two areas that you mentioned. Every pound of lean-body tissue that you gain will result in an additional 20 to 30 calories per day that will be "burned off." Just a five-pound gain in lean-body mass will result in a loss of about one pound of fat every month—or *twelve pounds of fat per year*!

Secondly, you have not indicated that you are doing any cardiovascular training as a regular part of your workout. Cardiovascular training will not only help to burn calories while you train—usually at a rate of about 5 to 15 calories per minute depending upon the intensity level of the exercise—but it will also allow you to strength train with a higher level of intensity which will engender greater gains. Doing just 30 minutes five times per week of moderate cardiovascular exercise (such as walking) will result in a fat loss of about one to three pounds of fat per month — or yet *another 12 to 36 pounds of fat per year*, depending upon your current metabolism and exercise intensity.

And as for the sit-ups, remember that THERE IS NO SUCH THING AS SPOT REDUCING! As plausible as it might seem, you could do hundreds of sit-ups per day and never significantly reduce the fat around your waist until you address the issue of fat loss through proper exercise and a sensible eating plan. Sit-ups are great for strengthening the abdomen—which has lots of health benefits—but don't expect the fat around your waist to melt away like butter in a pan. You must burn off more calories than you consume before fat loss will occur.

What is the best activity to do if I just want to lose weight?

What you are really saying is that you want to lose fat. And fat loss is still a question of calories *in* versus calories *out*. The best activity for virtually anyone who has been sedentary for an extended period of time is brisk walking. Please notice that I said BRISK walking (at least 3½ to 4 miles per hour) since the amount of distance covered during a specific time frame is, of course, directly related to speed. Although walking in and of itself is certainly better than remaining sedentary, an attempt should be made to make the walking workout rise to a level of at least *moderate* intensity. A speed of 3½ miles per hour (mph) means that a mile is completed in a little more than 17 minutes. At 4 mph, a mile is completed every 15 minutes. An average person can "burn" about 150 calories every 30 minutes at that speed. A one-hour walk will burn about 300 calories at that same speed. Accomplished every day, the result is nearly a three-pound loss of fat per month. That's more than 30 pounds of fat loss in one year by just adding this simple activity to your daily routine.

If you don't have time to walk for one hour every day, the good news is that the walking time can be divided up throughout the day. For example, a 30-minute walk at lunch time and another 30-minute walk after dinner can still produce the same caloric expenditure and achieve the same result. Many find that, after a while, walking briskly is not as challenging as it once was and slow jogging or running takes its place. Of course, with increased speed during the same time frame even more calories are burned and the fat loss is even greater. Studies have also shown that a regular walking program will not only help to reduce fat levels in the body but will also assist in lowering levels of the "bad" cholesterol known as LDL's (low-density lipoproteins).

Remember that it's okay to start out slowly and gradually increase the speed at which you walk. As the body becomes more fit, gradually increase the speed or the distance and you'll find that you have a new fitness and weight management program that's easy to do and easy to fit into your schedule. After all, walking can be done almost anywhere and at almost anytime. And don't forget the contribution that a comprehensive strength training program can play in changing your body composition.

I never seem to be able to lose weight and I gain weight very easily. Am I one of those people who is destined to be over weight or fat for the rest of my life?

Everyone has a choice in what they want to become. Although it is true that about 2% of the population has a biological reason (generally glandular) for being overweight or obese, 98% of the population has an opportunity to manage their weight through exercise and a reasonable eating plan. Only your doctor can determine if you are in the first category and the chances are very good that you are in the second category. Clearly, genetics do play a role in how easily we can manage our weight and, therefore, some individuals such as yourself MAY need to be somewhat more vigilant in living a healthy lifestyle. But it all gets down to a question of degree of commitment to being as fit as you can be. Not everyone can be slender and "toned". Not everyone can lose fat weight quickly and easily. But the formula for optimizing our genetic potential is nearly the same for everyone. And regular moderate levels of exercise is a major ingredient to *long-term* success.

For example, losing just 10% of your fat weight (for example, reducing your percentage of body fat from 25% to 22½%) can significantly reduce your chances of suffering from a variety of diseases such as heart disease, some types of cancer and even diabetes. This type of moderate fat loss will also result in a greater level of energy as well as an improved ability to engage in moderate exercise. As always, EXERCISE IS MEDICINE! It is the simplest and least expensive form of disease prevention that we have. And exercise doesn't have to be brutal or grueling. In fact, moderate levels of exercise—any exercise—accomplished over the *long-term* is the smart way to get fit and stay fit.

The next two chapters will address goal setting and some simple methods of measuring progress as well as ways of keeping your exercise routine sufficiently intense to produce the results that will assist in any weight management program.

Chapter Two
Goal Setting and Measuring Progress

One of the main reasons that workout programs fail is that people expect too much too soon. After a decade of neglect, it's not unusual for an individual to expect rapid weight loss and firm, "toned" muscles in four to six weeks. When the results don't happen as quickly as is desired, interest is lost and the program is abandoned. Or even more frequently, too much exercise is attempted too early in the program and, with sore and aching muscles and a deflated sense of accomplishment, the individual, who just a few days or weeks earlier was brimming with enthusiasm, quits their program and feels that they are doomed to failure. Sound familiar? Well, it happens all the time. If you are reading this book, it has probably happened to you—maybe even more than once.

I suppose that this is why "fad diets" are so popular. Just eat a specific amount or type of food or deny yourself a specific amount or type of food and you'll look like a million. And "dieting" is something that can be accomplished while sitting still with no exercise required. What could be easier than that, right?? Well, the sad truth is that both of these approaches to weight management and fitness improvement are all too common and, nearly always, grimly unsuccessful. More on "diets" in Chapter Four, but understand that the underlying reason for the failed programs described above are directly related to inaccurate program feedback and measurement. In other words, we can't or won't stay motivated unless we can see, on a regular and frequent basis, that we are actually progressing, improving or getting better.

GOAL SETTING

John F. Kennedy, in his inaugural address in January of 1961 said, "A journey of 1,000 miles begins with the first step, so let us begin." Setting fitness goals is not much different. It doesn't mean that we have to go 1,000 miles (although given the proper time and motivation, we just may) but it does mean that one of the most important aspects of a fitness program is just getting started. And this means that we need to set goals that are *reasonable and achievable* while maintaining a view of the big picture.

As mentioned earlier, most individuals begin a fitness program with weight management (fat loss) as their major goal. Hopefully, improved strength, endurance and flexibility are also included as program goals for reasons that were discussed in Chapter One. But most are looking for a way of transforming or changing the body to a preconceived notion of what it should, can or used to look like. And this is usually where the challenge begins. Setting a reasonable long-term goal is the first step in creating and, more importantly, maintaining a fitness program that will represent a permanent part of one's lifestyle. Understanding the true objective, however, is just as important.

For example, almost everyone will tell you that they exercise or need to exercise to "stay in shape" or to "get fit." Although these goals are seemingly correct, they are also somewhat nebulous or difficult to grasp unless certain factors are measured and used as feedback for future workouts and program modifications. "Staying in shape" or "getting fit" may mean different things to different people and many programs fail because the parameters that will represent success are never defined or, as mentioned, measured accurately. Cardiovascular training may result in improved endurance and stamina. It may also mean a lowered blood-pressure measurement, a reduction in stress, a higher caloric expenditure (which results in greater fat loss), the improved ability to walk, run, bike, hike or even swim a specific distance, or even lowering one's cholesterol. All of these "goals" may be attempted specifically or generally but they can all be measured to provide feedback and, therefore, motivation to continue training.

Without measurement on a regular and scheduled basis, the effort required to participate in a regular program of fitness as a part of one's lifestyle becomes more difficult. For example, it is well known that regular cardiovascular training can accomplish all of the goals listed previously. The exerciser, however, must make the effort to regularly measure these parameters as an integral part of his or her program. For example, going for a walk or a run as part of a cardiovascular fitness program is far more effective and motivational if just a few simple items are measured and compared. Instead of just "going out and walking" or "going for a run," measure or know the distance covered, keep track of the time spent during the activity and, most importantly, keep an accurate record of the heart rate. Chapter Three will provide more information on this topic as well as simple written workout recording devices to help keep you on track.

THE PHASES OF TRAINING

The real secret, however, to achieving long-term goals is to learn to break them down into a series of short-term goals that are reachable within a specific and reasonable period of time. Indeed, most fitness programs can be easily broken down into three simple phases. These phases can be further broken down into specific time frames or "mini-goals" that will assist in providing the feedback necessary to inform the participant and keep them excited about further progress. The three basic stages are known as the initial phase, the improvement phase and the maintenance phase.

The Initial Phase

The initial phase is probably the most critical because it is during this four to eight week period that many individuals give up. The main reason for this failure rate is that the participant starts out far too aggressively in pursuit of the long-term goal. For example, a person wishing to lose 25 pounds during this initial phase is likely to be disappointed and to consider the program a failure. Generally, because progress is perceived as too slow, more and more exercise at higher and higher levels of intensity are added until the program becomes difficult to maintain due to its vigorous and physically stressful content. The result is likely to be "non-compliance" which is a technical term for "I quit and I don't want to do this anymore." Understanding that it is during this initial phase that the groundwork for preparing the body progressively for a long-term commitment to exercise is a positive step in staying or "complying" with the program.

In the example above, a short-term goal of losing 10 pounds in the first month (just 2½ pounds per week) of the original long-term goal of 25 pounds would ultimately result in a more motivated individual who has an easier time accepting, understanding and even enjoying their program due to the smaller but still positive progress that was made. Intensity levels during the initial phase are generally kept low and the frequency and time frames for exercise should be monitored on a workout-by-workout basis. Of course, body-composition measurements (to be discussed in Chapter Five) would also be a part of the information provided as feedback. Appendix B and J described in Chapter Three will provide simple recording mechanisms for tracking and documenting both cardiovascular and strength training workouts.

The Improvement Phase

The second phase, the improvement phase, generally lasts from as little as four weeks to as long as six months. With the body better prepared to accept a slightly and progressively higher level of intensity, even more progress can be made, measured and recorded. For example, it would not be unusual for the resting heart rate (a simple measure of general fitness) to be reduced from an average of 72 beats per minute to, perhaps, 65 or 66 beats per minute (an improvement of about 10%) during the improvement phase. Indeed, it is quite possible that this improvement began during the initial phase and continued during the improvement phase.

The Maintenance Phase

The final phase, known as the maintenance phase, is reached when an initial and pre-established long-term goal has been accomplished. If a weight-loss goal has still not been reached after approximately six months, it is a good idea at this juncture to reassess and reset another series of short-term and long-term goals. It should be kept in mind that after approximately six months, both short-term and long-term goals for the next six months MAY be somewhat harder to reach as compared to the initial six months of the program. Weekly and monthly goals may need to be modified so that they remain challenging yet reasonable and *reachable*! Since the sometimes rapid improvements experienced during the initial phase and improvement phase have slowed somewhat, caution must be taken to realistically evaluate the goals for the next 6 months. This deceleration of improvement is true for strength training as well and Chapter Three will provide some helpful information in this regard.

Periodic evaluations of progress, whether it involves blood-pressure reduction, improved resting heart rate, strength levels or any other pre-established or desired goal, should be a regular part of any fitness program. After all, stupidity has been defined as doing the same thing over and over again and expecting different results. Even a fitness routine can occasionally benefit from a slight tune-up.

MEASURING PROGRESS

Appendices B, C and J provide workout recording sheets that includes the information that will help to accurately measure progress and provide feedback for short-term and long-term program modifications. Described in detail in Chapter Three, they provide areas for the participant to list all of the important information for every cardiovascular and strength training workout as well as body composition and flexibility measurements. They can be copied and, therefore, used over and over again. As you can see, and as discussed in the next chapter, all that is required for cardiovascular training is a measured distance and an accurate watch that measures minutes and seconds in order to take most of the necessary measurements that are needed to accurately assess your progress.

Girth measurements are described and a recording sheet is shown in Appendix C and an area for recording body-composition measurements (described and discussed in Chapter Five) is also provided. Directions for the completion of a simple flexibility test (The Sit and Reach Test) are also provided at the bottom of Appendix C. A space to record the results is also given.

Frequently Asked Questions

What is considered a reasonable weight-loss goal?

There is a considerable amount of evidence to suggest that those individuals who lose more than 2 to 2½ pounds per week are far more likely to gain back the weight than those who lose the weight at a more moderate rate over time. The reason is that when body weight is lost rapidly, the weight that is shed is not all fat weight. Indeed, it is possible that a significant proportion of the weight is lean-body tissue. Since lean-body tissue has a metabolic component (in other words, a loss of lean tissue means that less calories are being burned on a regular basis), additional body weight is easily regained if the individual's "diet" is not adhered to in a strict manner. This is another reason why proper eating plans (to be discussed in Chapter Four) are so important to success.

But let's face it, at a rate of 2 to 2½ pounds per week, it is possible to lose 8 to 10 pounds per month. That's more than 100 POUNDS PER YEAR! Most individuals who are significantly overweight would consider that amount of weight loss a tremendously successful program. For most individuals who feel they are carrying around an extra 15 or 20 pounds, an 8- to 10-week program would be sufficient. Of course, it would be hoped that any individual who reaches a desired weight goal would continue to participate in a regular program of exercise and proper eating so that it becomes a part of their lifestyle. Chapter Five will present and discuss methodologies for measuring and assessing fat weight versus lean-body mass.

The real key, however, is to be patient and accept moderate yet regular progress, particularly in the case of weight loss. In most cases being "overweight" (increased level of fat) is caused by months and, perhaps, years of bad habits and/or neglect. Expecting the situation to be resolved in a few days or even a few weeks is an unrealistic attitude that will frequently result in frustration and failure. It IS possible to lose fat weight permanently with a few simple changes in lifestyle but it takes time in order to be done right. Quick fixes are generally not a recipe for success particularly for the long-term.

What tests should be done by a doctor?

As mentioned in Chapter One, a doctor can help to determine if there are any physical complications that may limit one's participation in an exercise program. Heart rate and blood pressure are the typical indicators of the fitness of the cardiovascular system and, if deemed appropriate, fitness tests such as a step test or a graded treadmill test may be administered. Some fitness centers also offer these same graded fitness tests. Chapter Three will describe the method for taking your own heart rate (both resting heart rate and training heart rate) and blood pressure kits are available for home use for a reasonable cost. Measuring body composition will be presented in Chapter Five so that you will be able to determine your body's level of fat weight and, more importantly, determine how much of your weight loss (or gain) is lean-body mass and how much is fat weight. Some of these body-composition tests should only be administered by a doctor or a trained professional such as a certified personal trainer or fitness assessment specialist for purposes of accuracy.

If my goal is to improve my endurance, how will I know if I have achieved it?

Other than your perception of your current level of fitness (in other words, you simply feel that you have greater endurance, energy or stamina), exercising heart rate and resting heart rate are good indications that your body has become more fit. As noted in Chapter One, the heart and circulatory system are the ways that your body delivers oxygen to the cells to produce energy.

Exercise heart rate, also known as "training heart rate", is the number of times per minute that your heart must beat in order to perform a specific exercise task (such as walking or running a mile). If you accomplished a specified exercise task with a heart rate that is lower than it was, say, a month earlier when you performed the same exercise task, you can be considered to have better endurance or to be in better condition. This is because more blood and, therefore, oxygen was delivered to the working cells in less beats per minute—an indication that the function of the heart and circulatory system has improved. Another indication of improved endurance or cardiovascular fitness is the "resting heart rate." A lowered resting heart rate, generally taken upon arising in the morning, can indicate that the oxygen-delivering capability of the heart and circulatory system has improved.

How do I know when to modify or change my program goals?

Whenever progress has leveled off or "plateaued," it is time to look at program content. Leveling off of performance is generally caused by too much or too little of a specific program factor. As you will find in the next chapter, exercise intensity can either be too little (not quite intense enough in terms of exercise effort or frequency) or too much (overexercising which causes the body to require more recovery time). The idea is to give the body only what it needs and not what it can tolerate. Just as too little exercise is not effective in producing measurable results, significantly higher levels of exercise, over time, may have the same result.

It is a good idea to review the general fitness plan every four to six weeks to determine which components are working and to, perhaps, redirect or revise components that don't seem to be working or that are, quite frankly, intolerable to maintain for the long-term. This is also why accurately measuring program components—such as heart rate, flexibility, body composition and strength—are so important in establishing or reestablishing short-term program goals that will provide more immediate feedback and produce the motivation to continue the fitness program as a part of one's lifestyle.

Is it necessary to document or record everything with respect to the workout content?

That depends upon the goals of the program and how easily and quickly you can learn to measure the results of each workout. As you'll see in Chapter Three, recording each strength training workout and "setting up" the next workout takes but a few seconds after each exercise (and a workout card is available that you can download and use over and over). For cardiovascular training (endurance) and for flexibility improvement, the measurements are easy to learn how to do and, again, can be recorded easily and quickly. It is this workout-by-workout information, especially as it pertains to strength and cardiovascular training, that provides a quick peek into one's progress and makes planning the next workout so simple. Flexibility training can be measured and evaluated every two or three weeks and body composition can be assessed each month or so. The fitness program review schedule is up to the individual and depends, in large part, upon how much feedback he or she needs to remain comfortable and excited about training to be or stay fit. It really is simple to do and without the information concerning progress, program adherence (i.e., sticking with it) becomes far more difficult over time. The appendices provide all of the workout measurement and recording information that you will need to get started or even restarted on a program that's just right for you. Many of the recording logs can be copied to use "as is" or downloaded as desired (see appendices for details). The measurements themselves can be easily done by yourself or, in the case of some of the body-composition elements that are done only periodically, by a fitness professional at a fitness center near you. Your doctor may also want to use some of the body composition measurements as a regular part of an annual check-up since body weight, as you already realize or will soon find out, is only part of the story of transforming and improving your body and your level of fitness. You may even want to bring your workout and fitness data with you on your next visit to your doctor.

Are there any devices that can be used at a typical fitness center that can measure fitness levels?

Yes, and the most common one for measuring cardiovascular fitness is a stationary bike. Many current models have heart-rate monitors built into the handgrips that can determine your work capacity after you have entered some very simple information such as your age and current weight. In addition, many treadmills and stepping machines also have this technology. Basically, the machine (bike, treadmill, etc.) automatically measures your workload and, with the heart-rate information from the handgrips, determines your oxygen consumption. Usually, this oxygen consumption is measured in what are known as METS or "metabolic equivalents." A single MET is 3.5 milliliters of oxygen per kilogram of body weight per minute and is equal to the amount of oxygen your body consumes while at rest. But before you dash for your calculator or decide that it's too complicated to figure out, simply record the METS from your most recent workout on any device that has this capability and use it as your base level. For example, 5.3 METS would equal 18.55 milliliters of oxygen per kilogram of body weight per minute(or simply ml/kg/min). Your goal for your next workout, of course, might be to accomplish the same workload at 5.4 METS or 18.90 ml/kg/min. Even if you don't improve with the next workout, you can at least dazzle your workout buddies with your new vocabulary. Seriously, establishing your base or starting level is just that easy. And if MET levels are too confusing, you can always rely on measuring and recording training heart rate response that we discussed earlier.

By setting reasonable and achievable short-term goals, the long-term goals seem to take care of themselves. Also, by keeping track of just a few simple bits of workout information as you complete your fitness program or activity each time that you participate (and there should be at least a little bit of activity each day), it is possible to be constantly engaged in and excited about your ability to improve your level of fitness and general health. As you have either seen or will soon see, this periodic (sometimes daily) reviewing of your progress is what will keep you coming back for just a little more each time. Understand that little victories achieved will, over time, produce the final result that you seek. Further understanding that it will take time and that fitness and improved health is a lifetime commitment, endeavor to enjoy the journey. Little setbacks will, and usually do, happen but this is what program modification is all about. Skipping a workout or eating too much of the wrong food does not mean that you have failed in your long-term attempt to be fit or stay fit. It simply means that it is time to refocus, review your results and set new goals.

My workout partner seems to make better and more regular progress in some areas than I do and we both seem to work out with equal intensity and frequency. Is there something wrong with my workout?

As noted in Chapter One, the best person to compare yourself to in terms of progress and results is yourself. There are many factors that determine how "quickly" or effectively that an individual can improve their fitness levels. Many of these factors are genetic. In Chapter Five, there is a brief description of the three major body "types" presented in the context that not everyone has the same potential for rate of fat loss or gain and rate of lean-body mass gain (the ability to gain muscle). Aside from these body "types," there are a few other factors that, by themselves or in combination, can have fairly significant effects on strength and fitness potentials and limitations. These largely genetic factors are limb length, muscle-fiber types and their distribution pattern throughout the body, hormonal influences and what is known as "innervation" patterns.

It is possible, for example, that when comparing strength levels by using a pressing movement such as a seated press or a bench press, longer arms could be considered a disadvantage because of the additional work that must be accomplished for each repetition that is completed (in other words, the resistance is being raised or lifted a greater distance with each repetition). An individual with shorter limbs would be able to lift a similar resistance with less work per repetition.

As for muscle-fiber types and their distribution, it should be realized that there are basically two major muscle-fiber types (although a few "subtypes" have been identified) that are distributed throughout the body. They are generically known as fast-twitch and slow-twitch muscle fibers. Fast-twitch fibers can be said to fatigue quickly and slow-twitch fibers can be said to fatigue somewhat more slowly. Fast-twitch fibers are considered to have greater potential for strength and power while slow-twitch fibers are known primarily for their endurance capabilities. Every individual has both types of these muscle fibers in DIFFERENT distributions throughout the body. It's one of the things that makes us all unique and helps to explain, perhaps, why some individuals are "naturally" strong and gain muscle mass easily while others who train just as hard have a more difficult time getting the results that they desire. This is also where realistic goal setting in terms of short-term and long-term results can help to avoid frustration and program failure.

Hormonal influences can also have an effect on fitness program success in the sense that certain individuals have naturally higher levels of testosterone (and yes, females do have small amounts of testosterone) or a variety of other hormones that affect the body's ability to grow and repair itself. Since these hormonal levels can be slightly different in every person, their influences may also produce slightly different results.

"Innervation" patterns refer to the body's ability to stimulate muscles to move. The muscles move in response to stimulation by what are known as "motor units." A motor unit is a nerve cell and all of the muscle fibers that the individual nerve "innervates" or causes to contract when "fired." There are millions and millions of these nerve cell generated motor units in the body. Some individuals seem to have more motor units that "fire" more muscle fibers into action while others seem to have less. This number and distribution of nerves and motor units is genetically determined and unchangeable—*trainable* but *unchangeable*.

As you can see, there are many reasons why individuals can respond differently to similarly intense and comprehensive training programs. But it's not a reason to think that everyone cannot improve his or her physical fitness levels to a degree that promotes greater health. So be careful of comparisons, they can be misleading and lead to frustration and confusion. Find your own level of fitness, work to improve it on a regular basis and let the genetic factors take care of themselves.

Chapter Three

Controlling Workout Intensity

There is never a shortage of individuals who have explained to me that they have started fitness programs in the past and have failed because "it just wasn't working" or "I wasn't getting the results that I wanted." In many cases, this failure was based on the inability to measure results accurately or, even more importantly, to understand when to increase or decrease workout intensity so that they were accomplishing something in a way that provided feedback on a regular basis. Even the simplest workouts or "exercise programs" such as walking can produce greater results and long-term program adherence if the content of the exercise or activity can be measured accurately and simply.

The concept of "exercise intensity" follows what is known as an upside down "J" curve in terms of training response (see Figure 3.1 on the following page). It seems natural that the harder that one trains or works out, the greater the return in terms of improved fitness levels—and for the most part this is true. What is not as well understood or accepted is that exercise does not have to be prolonged or even significantly intense in order to produce a "training effect" which is generally defined as an improvement of one or more measures of fitness, usually endurance and/or strength.

Indeed, many exercisers—both beginners and experienced exercisers—feel that if the workout or fitness routine is not somewhat torturous, it is not effective. As one can easily see in Figure 3.1, there is a general improvement in the body's response to exercise as the exercise becomes more intense. But as one can also see, there can be a diminishing return when an individual reaches a certain level of intensity in terms of a lack of progress which is usually caused by a lack of proper recovery time (i.e., overtraining) and an increased incidence of injury.

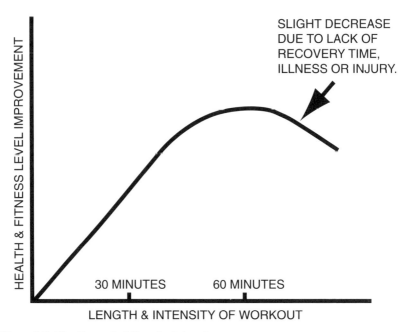

Figure 3.1: The Concept of Exercise intensity

Clearly, a workout or exercise routine needs to be challenging to some degree. The idea, of course, is to challenge the body and its circulatory system (heart, blood, arteries and veins), respiratory system (the lungs and oxygenated blood supply) and/or the muscoloskeletal system (the muscles, tendons, ligaments and the bones to which they are attached) by gradually pushing it up to and slightly beyond its current level of capability. And it is this "gradual" progress that many find so hard to define and, perhaps, control. But any small amount of progress, if it can be measured and recorded, can provide not only valuable feedback as to current progress but can also act as an instant motivational tool that can improve long-term exercise adherence. And it is progress over the long-term that is the real secret to a successful fitness program for each individual.

So what are the parameters that need to be measured, particularly with respect to cardiovascular training (training the heart, lungs and circulatory system) and strength training? Let's take a look at each one in more detail to determine a proper and optimal level of intensity for YOU!

First, if you are attempting to exercise for the first time or if you have been sedentary for an extended period of time, please review the PAR-Q provided in Appendix A. Indeed, this is a good idea even if you are a regular exerciser. Additionally, if you are a male over 35 years of age or a female over 40 years of age, it is recommended that you see your doctor before beginning any exercise program. This is especially true if you have a history of heart or circulatory problems or if these problems are common in your family.

Please note that if your health and fitness profile change so that you answer YES to any of the PAR-Q questions, tell your fitness or health professional. Ask them whether or not you should change your physical activity plan.

CARDIOVASCULAR TRAINING

When attempting to improve endurance, it is the cardiovascular system that is generally targeted as the key to improvement in this regard. Chapter One described and explained this system in a little more detail, but suffice it to say that wherever there is an improvement in the fitness level of the heart and lungs, there is a concomitant improvement in endurance. And this improvement is generally measured by the ability of the body to deliver oxygen to the cells for the production of energy. The more oxygen that is delivered to the cells, the more energy that can be produced. Therefore, in order to train the heart, lungs and circulatory system, they must be gradually and progressively challenged by exercise. Cardiovascular exercise is generally considered activities that involves large muscle groups that are moved rhythmically and/or repeatedly for a sustained period. Common cardiovascular activities include walking, running, biking and swimming.

And the initial level of challenge (especially for the new exercisers) does not have to be significant or difficult to be effective. Basically, the idea is to measure three different parameters or "things" in order to chart progress and measure improvement. Those three things are: time (the time it takes to complete the exercise bout), distance (or workload) and heart rate. For example, a brisk walk can be a great activity (especially for new exercisers) because it is relatively easy to measure the distance covered and the time taken to complete the distance. It is also easy to measure heart rate to determine if the exercise (in this case walking) is challenging the heart and circulatory system to deliver more oxygenated blood to the body to help produce the energy necessary to complete the task.

You can measure your heart rate by taking either your carotid or radial pulse. (See accompanying photographs.) To determine the beats per minute, simply count the number of beats for ten seconds and multiply the number by six or count the number of beats for 15 seconds and multiply the number by four.

Appendix B illustrates the cardio training log that can be copied and used to record activities and the intensity levels for those activities so that performance and progress can be easily charted. But before the content and recording of a sample workout is explained, let's review the "training heart rate" formula explained in Chapter One. As you recall, the "training heart rate" (THR) or "target heart rate" can be determined in two ways. One method to determine the age-predicted maximum heart rate using is the formula 220 – Age. A percentage of this

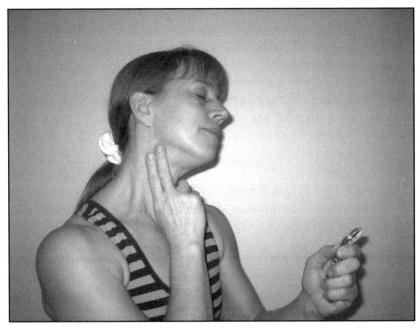

Carotid Pulse: *To take the carotid pulse, place the fingertips, as shown above, on the neck just to the side of the windpipe (larynx).*

maximum heart rate is used as the training heart rate. For beginners, this can be as low as 50 to 60% of the age-predicted maximum heart rate. Regular exercisers may be able to accomplish 60 to 80% of their age-predicted maximum and competitive athletes may choose to tolerate even higher levels when preparing for competition. Let's look at an example!

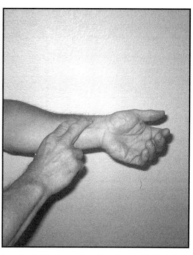

If a 40-year-old man (Joe) and woman (Susan) wish to begin a walking program to improve their fitness level, their maximum heart rate would be considered to be 180 beats per

Radial Pulse: To take the radial pulse, place the fingertips, as shown, on the wrist about an inch below the base of the thumb.

minute (220 – 40 = 180 beats per minute). Since they are beginners or inexperienced exercisers, they have chosen 60 to 70% of the age-predicted maximum (108 beats per minute to 126 beats per minute) as their "training heart rate." They have decided to walk for 20 minutes a day for the first two weeks of their program. They have determined that they can cover 0.6 miles on their first workout by walking around their neighborhood for 10 minutes and then returning by the same route and measuring the initial distance with their car odometer. They took their heart rate at the end of their walk Joe counted 18 beats in 10 seconds which means his heart rate was 108 beats per minute. Susan counted 19 beats in 10 seconds which means that her heart rate was 114 beats per minute. This means that they have reached their target or desired "training heart rate." On their card, they would record the activity (walking), the time (20 minutes), the distance completed and their heart rates.

The next time that Joe and Susan take their walk, they now have what is known as a "base level" of performance for that particular activity. They can now compare the results of each workout to determine if they are improving or if a higher or lower intensity level is necessary. The same procedure would be

Cardio Training Log				
Activity/Date	10/04	10/06	10/07	10/09
Walking *Time:*	20 MIN	20 MIN	20 MIN	20 MIN
Distance or Workload	1.2 MI	1.2 MI	1.2 MI	1.25 MI
Heart Rate	108 BPM	102 BPM	98 BPM	92 BPM
Brisk Walking *Time:*				
Distance or Workload				
Heart Rate				
Running *Time:*				
Distance or Workload				
Heart Rate				
Rowing *Time:*				
Distance or Workload				
Heart Rate				
Swimming *Time:*				
Distance or Workload				
Heart Rate				
Step Machine *Time:*				
Distance or Workload				
Heart Rate				
Elliptical Trainer *Time:*				
Distance or Workload				
Heart Rate				
Stationary Bike *Time:*				
Distance or Workload				
Heart Rate				
Biking *Time:*				
Distance or Workload				
Heart Rate				
Other *Time:*				
Distance or Workload				
Heart Rate				

Figure 3.2: Use of the Cardio Training Log

used regardless of the cardiovascular or "aerobic" activity that would be chosen. On their next 20-minute walk, in which they complete the same distance of 1.2 miles, they discover that their heart rates have dropped slightly. Joe shows a heart rate response to the "workout" of 102 beats per minute and Susan shows a heart rate response of 108 beats per minute. This means that each of them has become more efficient at delivering oxygen to their cells in response to the "workload" (the 20-minute walk) since their hearts had to beat a few less times per minute to accomplish the same task. As a result, it is likely over time that their resting heart rates will also be lowered, yet another sign of improved cardiovascular fitness. This concept—and that of how to record workout data—is illustrated in Figure 3.2.

After the first week or two of their new walking program, Joe and Susan will find it necessary to gradually increase the intensity level of their workout. This will be needed because their hearts and circulatory systems will progressively become more efficient and the 1.2 miles in 20 minutes will become less and less challenging. At this point, they will determine which parameter or workout variable will be changed in order to continue to gently and effectively challenge their bodies to improve. They can either increase the time that they spend doing the activity, increase the speed at which they walk or they can do both. The determining factor that will drive their decision will more than likely be what is known as "perceived exertion" — the second method of measuring workout intensity.

Perceived exertion is a method that involves rating one's intensity (or exertion) level on a scale of 1 to 10. Previously, the scale commonly used (known as the Borg Scale of Perceived Exertion) involved ratings from 6 to 20. Both are useful. However, using a scale of 1 to 10 is generally considered somewhat easier to do. (Figure 3.3 shows a modified perceived exertion scale.) Generally, a perceived exertion level of 3 or 4 on a scale of 1 to 10 is considered as a moderate level of exercise with the 1 representing a low level of exertion such as sitting still and 10 representing an exertion level of extreme difficulty or effort that is difficult to maintain for an extended period of time. By exercising at a level of 3 or 4, it is common that the individual would be exerting themselves at a level that would produce a moder-

Rating	Perceived Exertion	Intensity
0	Nothing at All	
0.5	Extremely Weak	Just Noticeable
1	Very Weak	
2	Weak	Light
3	Moderate	Light to Medium
4		Medium to Heavy
5	Strong	Heavy
6		
7	Very Strong	Very Heavy
8		
9		
10	Extremely Strong	Strongest

Figure 3.3: Modified Perceived Exertion Scale

ate training effect and a heart-rate response approximating 60 to 70% of their age-predicted maximum. Of course, it is a good idea to monitor the heart rate as well as the perceived exertion for reasons of safety since perceptions of exertion can be different for different people.

Another way of determining moderate levels of exertion for cardiovascular training is by taking what is known as the "talk test." With a moderate level of exertion, the exerciser is capable of carrying on a conversation while exercising. If the breathing is labored as a result of the exercise, it becomes more difficult to speak conversationally and the exercise intensity has likely exceeded the moderate range. A simple heart rate check would be in order if this is the case and it is also likely that the heart-rate response has exceeded 60 to 70% of the age-predicted maximum. Although this increased intensity can produce a greater training effect, it is more difficult for most individuals to sustain this level for extended periods of time. And it is for this reason that many people quit exercising aerobically. Again, more moderate levels of exercise over a longer period of time will generally produce greater program adherence and more frequent and steady improvement in cardiovascular fitness. But let's get back to Joe and Susan!

As a result of a lowered heart-rate response to their walking program (in other words, they are now a little more fit), they must decide to increase the intensity of their program to ensure continued improvement. Since their perceived exertion was considered to be a 4 on a scale of 1 to 10, let's assume that they have decided to increase the length of time that they walk while walking at the same rate of speed. Therefore, they decide to increase their walking *time* by 20 more minutes. Since they are enjoying the activity, they feel that this is easily possible and will, of course, monitor and record their heart rates to see if it remains or falls below their training heart rate zone of 60 to 70% of their age-predicted maximum. Eventually, after a few more weeks, it is likely that they will opt to increase their walking *speed* as they become more conditioned to the workout routine. This means that they will be walking farther and faster as they become more fit. It also means that they will be burning even more calories because they are exercising for a longer period of time and, eventually, at a higher intensity level.

As they continue to monitor their heart-rate response, they will probably notice that the level of walking that they can accomplish in terms of distance and speed will improve and that their heart-rate response will also continue to improve (in other words, it will be lower) as they become more fit. The improvement in their fitness is due to an improved ability of their hearts and circulatory systems to deliver more oxygen via the blood to their cells. It is this type of simple and long-term improvement that is the pattern for almost any type of cardiovascular exercise regardless of current levels of fitness. By measuring three simple parameters or variables (distance, speed and heart rate) and adjusting them based upon heart-rate response and perceived exertion, anyone can get started on a program of improved cardiovascular fitness. Whether the exercise of choice is walking, running, biking, swimming or any number or other "aerobic" activities, the method and progression is similar.

STRENGTH TRAINING

Probably no other area of fitness is more misunderstood than strength training. Understanding how much is too much or even how much is enough has likely been the main reason for more failed programs than any other factors. Fortunately, the answers are really quite simple and are based more on proper technique and accurate measurement than on "free weights" versus machines or grunt-and-groan contests on the much revered bench press. Indeed, every resistance modality has advantages and disadvantages. The real key, of course, is how they are used. There are plenty of home workout weight machines that become nothing more than expensive coat racks. And there are plenty of individuals wandering around fitness centers and gyms doing set after set of relatively meaningless exercise because they don't have an organized plan—or perhaps even a clue.

This section of the chapter on understanding intensity will focus largely on strength training technique and an understanding of the variables that can be used to personalize a total strength program for any individual regardless of experience or background. The principles are based upon safety and time management and represent a methodology for improving strength in an effective, organized and measurable way. The principles and variables are simple and, if followed carefully, will produce regular improvements in strength as well as in joint range of motion.

Since proper technique is important to a successful strength training program, we will begin with the recognized principles of a properly performed resistance exercise. These basic tenets of strength training will, in the absence of muscular disease, produce strength gains on a regular basis while helping to prevent overuse injuries and musculoskeletal problems associated with improper technique.

Principles of a Properly Performed Exercise

1. **Excercise through a Full Range of Motion**. Always lift the weight or resistance through a full "range of motion." This means that there can be no "cheating" or incomplete movement patterns. It is far better to lift less resistance through a complete range of motion than to lift a level of resistance that requires a reduced range of mo-

tion. This more careful and complete method will also promote flexibility as well as strength. A greater level of strength that can be demonstrated through an increased range of motion as a result of full range of motion exercise will produce stronger movement patterns and less injury-prone joints.

2. **Move the Weight or Resistance with Control**. Reduce momentum from the lifting technique to ensure that only the muscles are raising the resistance and that momentum is not a factor in the success of the completed repetition. By raising resistance using a controlled pattern, it is more likely that the resistance was lifted as a result of muscular work. Many individuals attempt to toss and "jerk" weights in order to lift more resistance. However, this not only makes it more difficult to accurately measure the workload, it could expose the joints and connective tissue to possible damage or injury. Additionally, these types of movements reduce the range of motion through which the resistance was lifted which may compromise flexibility. (See #1.) It is recommended that the resistance always be raised in a controlled manner which generally translates into a one- to two-second upward movement.

3. **Emphasize the Lowering of the Weight or Resistance**. Add greater intensity to each repetition by emphasizing the lowering of the weight as well as the controlled raising of the weight. It takes the same muscle to lower a weight or resistance against gravity as it does to raise the same resistance against gravity. However, since the resistance has already been raised, the lowering movement must be somewhat slower (usually two to four seconds) than the raising or upward movement in order for muscular work to be accomplished during the lowering phase. In this way, more work is accomplished per repetition than by only raising the weight. In addition, by emphasizing the lowering of the weight with each repetition, it is possible to challenge the muscle while using less weight due to the greater workload accomplished with each repetition.

4. **Challenge the Muscles**. Attempting to reach momentary muscular fatigue or what is also known as "volitional failure" is the only way to assure that the muscles involved in the movement have been recruited maximally. This means that by using a resistance that will produce fatigue or near-fatigue within a specific repetition range will assure that the maximum amount of work has been accomplished and can be recorded. This gives the exerciser an exact level of performance with a specific amount of resistance that can be used to gauge progress or determine the workload or resistance level for the next workout. (The specific suggested repetition ranges will be listed in the Q&A section focusing on exercise variables.)

5. **Supervision and/or "Partnering."** Whenever possible, strength train with a partner. This will not only help to improve the intensity of the exercise or lift (since we have a tendency to work harder when someone is watching), but it allows the strength trainer to receive constant coaching as to form as well as receiving a little bit more motivation. Training with a partner also has a tendency to improve long-term program compliance because we are more likely to *work out* on a regular basis when there is someone to *train with* on a regular basis. Lastly, the safety of the program will be enhanced since the training partner can assist in "spotting" on exercises that may be particularly challenging.

As you can see, there is a great deal of emphasis on strength training form. In order for the results of each set of exercise or each repetition of exercise to be an accurate measurement or assessment of strength at each subsequent workout, the technique used for each lift or exercise must be the same and must represent a true picture of the ability of the muscle(s) to overcome the resistance. But there are other factors that must be considered so that optimal levels of training can be accomplished. These factors are every bit as important as the basic principles of a properly performed exercise that have just been presented here. And they relate in a similar way to the FITT Principle (frequency, intensity, time and type) described in the section on the cardiovascular components of fitness in Chapter One. They will be presented here in the form of common questions concerning strength training variables that often confound and/or limit performance and progress in a poorly focused and poorly organized strength training program.

RESISTANCE EXERCISE VARIABLES

There are eight variables in organizing a program of resistance exercise repetitions, sets, duration, resistance, progression, frequency, sequence and volume. These variables will be discussed in a question and answer format.

How many repetitions should be performed?

For most individuals, it is recommended that 8 to 12 repetitions of each exercise WITH PROPER FORM be performed to volitional failure for upper body exercises, and 10 to 15 repetitions for the lower body. This means that if the individual chooses a resistance for the upper body where less than 8 repetitions are possible, the resistance is probably a little too heavy. Conversely, if more than 12 repetitions can be accomplished, the resistance is probably too light. For the lower body, the 10 to 15 repetition parameter should be used. Two or three workouts may be required in order to accurately determine the correct resistance level that will produce the desired number of repetitions. For beginners, a repetition range of 10 to 15 for the upper body muscles may prove helpful for the first few weeks, and 15-20 repetitions for the muscles of the lower body may be desirable initially.

How many sets should be performed?

For most individuals, it is recommended that one to three sets of each exercise and/or lift be performed. However, it should be noted that there is little scientific evidence to suggest that more than one set OF SUFFICIENT INTENSITY is significantly more effective than multiple sets. In either case, only the *first* set of exercise should be recorded on the strength training workout card. A simple, safe, brief and effective multiple-set system known as the Quick Set System will be presented in the next section.

How much time should I take in between each set of exercise?

As little time as possible should be taken in between sets of exercise. For beginners, this should be based upon "perceived exertion."

How much weight or resistance should be lifted?

The individual should determine how much resistance can be lifted WITH PROPER FORM in order to reach volitional failure within a range of 8 to 12 repetitions for the upper body muscles and 10 to 15 repetitions for the lower body. If the resistance can be lifted for more than 12 repetitions or 15 repetitions respectively (upper and lower body), the resistance should be increased, if possible, by about one or two percent. If less than 8 repetitions (upper body) or 10 repetitions (lower body) can be accomplished, the resistance should be reduced until the repetitions can be completed WITH PROPER FORM within the suggested range. Reminder: For beginners, a repetition range of 10 to 15 repetitions may prove helpful for the upper body for the first few weeks, and 15 to 20 repetitions for the muscles of the lower body may be easier to establish.

When should I increase the weight or resistance?

When more than 12 repetitions (upper body) or 15 repetitions (lower body) on the first set can be performed, it is time to increase the resistance for the next workout by one or two percent.

How often should a workout take place?

Since exercise recovery is an important factor in strength training response, it is recommended that workouts of adequate intensity be separated by 48 to 72 hours (about two or three days). For example, strength training on Monday, Wednesday and Friday would probably provide sufficient recovery time for workouts of adequate intensity.

Is there an optimal exercise order?

Most definitely! It is always a good idea to train the larger muscles first and "work down" to the smaller muscles. In this manner, larger muscle groups (such as the chest and upper back) are not limited by the "prefatiguing" of the smaller muscle groups (such as the arms) in exercises or lifts that use multiple muscle groups such as the bench press or "lat pulldown."

How many exercises or lifts should be done?

By accomplishing one lift or exercise for each of the major muscle groups in the body, it is possible for an experienced strength trainer to train the entire body in 30 to 40 minutes. For beginners, this time frame may be somewhat different depending upon their "perceived exertion" and how many exercises and/or lifts are included in their initial program. The Quick Set System (described next) will explain how this type of time efficient workout can be accomplished. The system can be used for virtually any exercise or lift in a total body program.

The Quick Set System

Many strength training programs fail because they are too daunting in terms of the number of exercises and sets. More importantly, they fail because most individuals feel that they simply don't have the time to complete a comprehensive workout in less than a couple of hours—or more. "Split routines," a method of training that involves working with specific body parts on specific days of the week, can be limiting because it allows the individual to train a certain body part only once or twice per week. Additionally, "split routines" require a daily trip to the fitness center or workout room and many people simply don't have the time to make this type of commitment on a regular basis. The result is a feeling of failure on the part of the exerciser and the long-term commitment to this aspect of the individual's comprehensive program is lost. The Quick Set System can help to solve this dilemma by allowing higher levels of training to be accomplished in a much shorter period of time. In addition, the intensity level of the workout *is increased* as the resistance used *is reduced*! This means that *less* resistance or weight is doing *more* work and the incidence of injury due to heavy resistance levels is also reduced.

The system involves only four simple steps and the results are easy to record on the strength training workout card in Appendix J. A sample of the recording method is shown for the chest press here in the text (p. 51) to assist in understanding both the method and how the results are recorded. But first, a recommendation for beginners or individuals who have been sedentary or inactive for an extended period of time.

As you recall, it is possible to obtain a "training effect" by accomplishing one set of resistance exercise provided that the exercise is completed to momentary failure or volitional fatigue within a specific number of repetitions (see Principles of a Properly Performed Exericise and Resistance Exercise Variables on pages 43-47). Since the Quick Set System is a training technique that involves a slightly higher level of intensity, it is recommended that the beginner or sedentary individual strength train using one set of properly performed exercise per body part for weeks one through three. During weeks four and five, a second set of exercise using the Quick Set System can be added. By week six, the complete system described next can be attempted. Now let's take a look at the Quick Set System.

How the Quick Set System Works

There are four easy steps to complete the system. It is a training method that is *safe*, *time efficient* and *effective* at delivering a sufficient level of intensity to any workout regardless of your current level of strength.

1. Determine the level of resistance that you can lift with proper form to muscular fatigue for 8 to 12 repetitions for any upper body exercise (i.e., muscle groups above the waist) and 10 to 15 repetitions for any lower body exercise (i.e., muscle groups below the waist).

2. When muscular fatigue is reached on the first set within the specified repetition range, immediately reduce the resistance or weight by approximately 25 to 30%. Begin lifting the reduced level of resistance as soon as possible and complete as many repetitions as possible with proper form. This will usually produce a set of approximately 6 to 10 repetitions with the lower weight. However, individual responses to this first "quick set" may vary quite a bit. Take as little time as possible in between sets.

3. When muscular or volitional fatigue on the second set (which is actually the first "quick set") is accomplished, repeat the process by reducing the resistance another 25

to 30%. Begin lifting as soon as possible with the reduced level of resistance. You will notice that even though the weight or resistance level on this third and final set is only about half that of the initial set of exercise, it is a level of resistance that is still challenging to the muscles. It is also a level of resistance that will optimize the training effect for that particular muscle group in only about three or four minutes or less.

4. Record the number of repetitions completed on the FIRST SET ONLY under the appropriate date on your workout card. Place the weight or resistance level above the slanted line and the number of repetitions below the slanted line (as shown in Figure 3.4). Fill in the resistance level for your next workout in advance. For example, if you exceeded the recommended number of repetitions for that body part, increase the resistance for your next workout accordingly. If you failed to reach the recommended number of repetitions, reduce the weight accordingly. In this manner, you will always have a new goal of either a slightly increased resistance level (if you surpass the recommended repetition range) or an increase in the number of repetitions that you will attempt to complete. It is this type of regular and accurate feedback that will help to keep you motivated to do a little more each time you strength train. Move on to the next strength training exercise! (Figure 3.5 shows a sample workout card.)

As you can see, the system is really quite simple and makes it easy to track results and set goals on a workout-by-workout basis. In this way, it is possible to get your entire strength training workout done in an efficient, safe and effective manner. You see, less weight really can do more work if you know the secret— the principles of properly performed exercise!

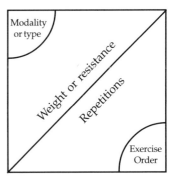

Figure 3.4:
How to Record Workout Data

BE FIT, STAY FIT!

BODY PART: Exercise/Lift	Month /Day				
CHEST: (2)					
* Chest Press/Bench Press 8-12 repetitions BB, M, DB					
Bent Arm Press 8-12 repetitions BB, M					
UPPER BACK: (2)					
Lat Pulldown 8-12 repetitions M					
* Seated Row 8-12 repetitions M					
Bent Over Row 8-12 repetitions DB					
Pullover 8-12 repetitions M					
SHOULDERS:					
Lateral Raise 8-12 repetitions DB, M					
* Seated Press 8-12 repetitions DB, BB, M					
Upright Row 8-12 repetitions BB					
HIPS:					
Squat 10-15, 15-20 repetitions BB					
* Leg Press 10-15, 15-20 repetitions M					
LEGS:					
* Leg Extension 10-15 repetitions M					
* Leg Curl 10-15 repetitions M					

50

BODY PART: Exercise/Lift					
LEGS (continued):					
Calf Raise **10-15 repetitions M**					
ARMS:					
Bicep Curl **8-12 repetitions DB, BB, M**					
Tricep Push Downs **8-12 repetitions M**					
ABS:					
Curl-ups					
Twisting Curl-ups					
OPTIONAL (Other Selected Exercises/Lifts):					
Example: Dips					

Modality Codes: BB= barbell, DB= dumbell, M= selectorized machine, Reps 8-12, 10-15, 15-20. Remember reminder to use the proper technique and to warm up and cool down before and after working out. The * designates items that are part of the core workout. A full page (8½ x 11) copy of this chart is available at www.cardinalpub.com/befit.

Sample

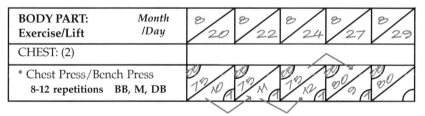

Figure 3.5: Workout Card with Sample Data. Notice the increase in weight or resistance and the increase in repetitions. On 8/29, note that the resistance is already recorded for the next workout.

FREQUENTLY ASKED QUESTIONS

I work out with weights and don't do much "cardio" training. Will that limit my progress or performance in the weight room?

An improved cardiovascular system should be part of any complete or comprehensive fitness program. The muscles require oxygen when they are being trained and if the cardiovascular system is functioning in an improved manner, this can mean even better performance in the strength training aspect of your program. In addition to providing more oxygen for the production of energy as a result of a stronger and more efficient heart, an improved cardiovascular system will increase capillary density (in other words more oxygen can be exchanged in the lungs and more oxygen can get to the working cells). Even more importantly, the mitochondria in your cells (the tiny engines of the cell) will increase in number as well as function more efficiently. This will result in greater available energy and muscle growth. So don't forget to make cardiovascular training a regular part of your overall program.

I've been running almost every day for months and I seem to have leveled off in my progress. What should I do?

There could be a number of reasons for the "leveling off" of your performance. First, I might recommend that you reduce the number of days per week that you run. This will allow you to, perhaps, recover from your running workouts a little more completely and allow your body some time to respond to the training stimulus of your workouts. Three to five days per week is considered optimal. If you feel that you must run EVERY day, then I would suggest that you reduce the time or distance of two or three of your weekly workouts to save the wear and tear on your body. You must remember that recovery time is every bit as important as the time spent training. It is during the recovery period(s) that the body responds, improves and regenerates.

Additionally, I would suggest that you include some strength training in your general program. A stronger musculoskeletal system will not only perform more efficiently, thereby saving energy, but it will also allow the body to recover from workouts more rapidly and, therefore, improve your running performance. And a stronger body will also reduce your chances of overuse injuries that are common to runners.

How do I know if I'm really in better "shape"?

Our culture has confused the word "shape" with the word "condition." An individual can appear to be in good "shape" because they seem to have good body proportions when, in actuality, they may be severely lacking in cardiorespiratory fitness and/or have little energy. Clearly, having acceptable body proportions is good in terms of not carrying around excess fat (a challenge shared by nearly half of all Americans) but being in good "condition" means that our bodies can produce energy easily and efficiently so that we can not only complete our jobs and daily tasks but have enough energy left over to participate in recreational activities and, in general, enjoy ourselves.

The best indicator of being in good "condition" is resting heart rate and the heart-rate response to exercise. Average resting heart rates for adult males and females are 72 BPM and 70 BPM respectively. It is possible, however, that an individual may have a resting heart rate that is average and still have a comparatively elevated heart rate when attempting to engage in simple activities such as walking. If this is the case, a progressive exercise program is in order so that the body can be gradually trained to respond to exercise with a lower heart-rate response which indicates that the cardiovascular system has improved its ability to deliver oxygen to the cells for the production of energy. In other words, the body can accomplish a greater workload with a lower heart rate response. For example, if you could run 2 miles in 20 minutes at a heart rate of 140 beats per minute three months ago and you can now run 2 miles in 19 minutes at a heart rate of 135 beats per minute, you have improved both the amount of work that you can perform as well as the efficiency of your heart and circulatory system as evidenced by your lowered heart rate. It is also likely that you have lowered your resting heart rate which is an indication of improved fitness as well.

Aside from heart-rate response, the other way that one can tell if they are in good shape is simply in the way they feel and the way that they perceive their body. Not everyone can have a perfect body or be in perfect condition all the time. But if one feels good, is energetic and is satisfied with how they look, they're probably on the right track in terms of their fitness levels.

Why are establishing "base levels" important?

Whether the subject is cardiovascular fitness, flexibility or strength fitness, you can't know how much or how well you have improved unless you have a good idea of where you started. And measuring your "base levels" or starting points is easy to do. As has already been shown, finding base levels for cardiovascular training is as easy as measuring distance (or workload), time and heart rate. Comparing performance on a regular basis, say weekly or monthly, will show if improvement has been accomplished.

For strength training, base levels are those levels of resistance or weight that are lifted with proper form within suggested or specified repetition ranges—generally these ranges are 8 to 12 for upper body exercises and 10 to 15 for lower body exercises. By recording the repetitions completed for the first set of each exercise done to momentary fatigue, it is possible to establish a base level and a goal for each exercise and for each workout. The goal, of course, is to do one or two more repetitions than the last time the exercise or lift was completed or to use a slightly higher resistance if the upper end of the suggested range has been reached consistently.

Chapter Four
Diet is a Four-Letter Word

You have probably noticed by now that each time I have used the word "diet" thus far in the book, I have placed it in quotation marks. This is because most people consider a diet as something that they "go on" for a brief period of time and then "go off" when they feel that a specific weight-loss goal has been achieved. Sad to say, most of those same people (nearly 90%) will regain most and sometimes even more of the weight that they lost while "dieting". That's because dieting is sort of like breathing through a straw. It's possible to do, it isn't necessarily pleasant and it is survivable BUT it is impossible to do forever. Diets simply don't work. Diets never have worked on a permanent basis and they never will work unless the word "diet" is perceived or defined differently.

A true diet (or eating plan) is what one eats on a regular basis all of the time and is a normal part of their everyday lifestyle. This also means, then, that is must be something that is acceptable, reasonable and, of course, palatable. The typical American view of a diet is nuts, seeds and twigs with a little low-calorie dressing three times a day. A "diet snack" is considered a dry rice cake. But the truth is that it is possible to eat many of the foods we love, in moderation of course, and still get the nutrients that we need to help make or keep our bodies healthy and fit. So from this point on I will use the terms "eating plan" and "diet" interchangeably so that they refer to the food that we are consuming every day. I'll even skip the quotation marks from now on when I use that four-letter word that we all know and love.

So how do we modify the diet so it's something that can be tolerated forever? How do we get all of the nutrients that we need without hunkering down over seaweed sandwiches and bok choy juice? The information that follows will, in general terms, present some guidelines and suggestions that should not only help to increase the "nutrient density" in our diets, it can and will help us to improve our fitness programs by taking in the nutrients necessary for our bodies to recover, grow and/or respond to our workouts more effectively. After all, a good exercise program and a lousy diet or eating plan is another reason why many fitness program fail. So let's see what's necessary to succeed.

I've already mentioned the term nutrient density and this term is an important one in attempting to create an effective eating plan with which one can live. Basically, it refers to the amount of a nutrient or nutrients in a food compared to the number of calories that it contains. For example, if an increased amount of calcium (a critical nutrient in the diet) is the goal, an 8-ounce glass of low-fat milk would be more nutrient dense than a scoop of ice cream. Both foods have about the same amount of calcium but the milk has fewer calories and a lower level of fat. That doesn't mean that ice cream does not have some nutrient value, but it does mean that one would probably want to choose the low-fat milk as a source of calcium more often than the ice cream. For those who might be lactose intolerant and, therefore, prefer low-fat yogurt to ice cream, it should be noted that low-fat yogurt has nearly twice the calories of low-fat milk. But the bottom line is that choices have to be made at nearly every turn and by using nutrient density as a method of increasing the intake while reducing the number of "empty" calories, anyone can improve their diet. And did you know that by eliminating just 200 "empty" calories per day, the average person can lose **20 pounds of fat per year!**

THE MAJOR NUTRIENTS

There are six major classes of nutrients that the body needs to stay healthy and fit. They are water, protein, carbohydrates, fats, vitamins and minerals. Only three of these classes of nutrients (proteins, carbohydrates and fats) contain calories. Proteins and carbohydrates contain 4 calories per gram while fats contain more than twice that number—9 calories per gram. It is the imbalance of these three classes of nutrients in the typical American diet that is considered one of the main reasons for the ever increasing levels of overweight and obesity in our culture.

Protein is, of course, an essential nutrient that helps to build and support muscle as well as other tissues in the body. It is recommended that the average person consume about 0.8 grams of protein per kilogram of body weight (that's about 0.4 grams per pound of body weight). For the average-size person, that's about 50 to 60 grams per day. The average American consumes around 100 grams of protein per day. In addition, the main sources of that protein are in the form of animal products. This means that they have a tendency to be higher in fat, and particularly saturated fat, than proteins from plant sources. As you can see, the challenge for the typical American, in terms of diet, is not from getting enough protein. Rather, it's consuming too much fat due to the food choices that are made as well as the serving sizes that are consumed.

For individuals who are involved in moderately or highly intense levels of fitness training, the amount of protein consumed MAY need to be increased to 1.0 to 1.2 grams or more of protein per kilogram of body weight. As one can easily deduce, the average American is still well within that guideline. So the question is not necessarily the amount of protein but the source of protein. Reducing the size of the portions of animal protein that are consumed daily to about one or two-four ounce servings and combining it or supplementing it with plant protein sources such as green vegetables, whole-grain products and beans is a simple way to get the protein that you need while reducing the consumption of fats (which, as you recall, has twice the calories per gram than does plant protein sources). Protein supplements are also a good source of protein with virtually no fat. Generally, protein should represent about 10 to 35% of the total calories consumed per day depending upon activity and training levels.

Carbohydrates should represent from 45 to 65% of the total calories that you consume and most of that should be in the form of "complex" carbohydrates—in other words, fruits and vegetables. Fruits and vegetables are extremely "nutrient dense" and, therefore, have a high content of various essential nutrients and, generally, are lower in calories. It is with these types of foods that many of the more than fifty essential micronutrients such as vitamins and minerals can be easily and regularly added to the diet. Additionally, carbohydrates are an excellent source of fiber. In fact, food listings on product packaging will usually list the fiber content of these foods. Higher fiber content in the diet has been associated with lower rates of heart disease and even some types of cancer such as colon cancer.

Even though fats have developed a bad name, they are an essential nutrient. Fats, or lipids, are an essential part of nearly every cell in the body, especially the cell membranes. Nerve cell membranes consist partly of these same lipids or fats. Fats also have a function as body insulators and even, in some cases, shock absorbers. Since fat has more than twice the calories per gram than proteins and carbohydrates, a daily diet high in fat will reach the saturation level of calories necessary to allow the body to function far more quickly. In other words, if the body needs 2,000 calories per day to function and perform necessary tasks, it will reach this level more rapidly if fat consumption is high. Since excess calories from any source—proteins, carbohydrates OR fats—are stored as body fat, it becomes easy to see why fats, though essential, should be limited. It is recommended that only 20 to 35% of the total calories consumed daily come from fat. The average American consumes a diet that is over 40% fat!

THE FOOD GUIDE PYRAMID

One of the easiest ways to make minor changes in the eating plan or diet that can have significant effect on fat loss and greater nutrient consumption is the Food Guide Pyramid shown in Figure 4.1. By comparing your current diet to the Food Guide Pyramid, it becomes easy to see where relatively minor adjustments

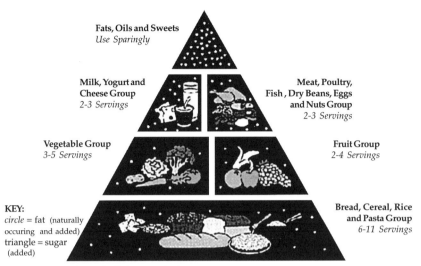

Figure 4.1: The Food Guide Pyramid

can be made in one's daily food choices. For many, comparing their diet to the suggestions shown on The Food Guide Pyramid can act as a wake-up call regarding how many "empty" or highly caloric foods they are eating.

How Many Servings Do You Need a Day?

	Women and Some Older Adults	Children, Teen Girls, Active Women, Most Men	Teen Boys and Active Men
Calorie level*	about 1600	about 2200	about 2800
Bread group	6	8	11
Vegetable group	3	4	5
Fruit group	2	3	4
Milk group	**2-3	**2-3	**2-3
Meat group	2, for a total of 5 ounces	2, for a total of 6 ounces	3, for a total of 7 ounces

* These are the calorie levels if you choose low-fat, lean foods from the 5 major food groups and use foods from the fats, oils, and sweets group sparingly.

** Women who are pregnant or breastfeeding, teenagers and young adults to age 24 need 3 servings.

Table 4.1: Suggested Daily Servings

ANALYZING YOUR CURRENT EATING PLAN

In order to compare your diet with that suggested by The Food Guide Pyramid, a simple Eating Plan Diary (EPD) has been provided in Appendix D. Appendix E shows the Eating Plan Analysis (EPA). Here's how it works: On the EPD, write down everything that you ate during a specific 24-hour period from the time that you arose to the time that you went to sleep. Choose the day randomly so that the results are more accurate. Remember to write down EVERYTHING that you ate or drank during that day no matter how insignificant it may seem. Appendix F illustrates and explains how to assess serving sizes and how to use the Food Guide Pyramid. Count your serving sizes appropriately since one serving of meat or poultry, for example, may actually need to be counted as two or three servings depending upon the size. Table 4.1 provides a list of suggested daily servings.

After you have written down everything that you have eaten for that day, compare your results with the EPA. Remember that servings from the meat group should be listed in total ounces rather than just the number of servings. On the right-hand side of your EPA, circle the appropriate box across from each food group. By this type of simple assessment, anyone can see where their diet or eating plan needs modification. In many cases, making minor adjustments in food intake can produce rapid and significant improvements in weight control, improved work-out performance and general health.

The Eight Key Nutrients

Now that you have compared your eating plan to the Food Guide Pyramid, you are ready to make the necessary changes that will increase or improve the nutrient density of your diet. But did you know that the five different food groups represented by The Food Guide Pyramid contain all of the eight key nutrients that will help you to ensure a balanced diet. It's true! By eating the foods in the quantities or amounts suggested in the Food Guide Pyramid, it is likely that you will consume the eight key nutrients and, at the same time, it is likely that you will also consume a sufficient supply of all the other nutrients that you need as well. Those key nutrients are: protein; vitamin A; three B-complex vitamins known as thiamin, riboflavin and niacin; vitamin C; iron and calcium. This does not mean that these key nutrients should be consumed only through supplementation. What it means is that if the balanced diet represented by the Food Guide Pyramid is consumed, these key nutrients will also be consumed. Moreover, those foods that contain these key nutrients will also contain most, if not all, of the other nutrients that are essential to good general health.

Ten Tips For Reducing Caloric Intake With Which You Can Live

1. **Reduce Portion Sizes.** Eating a six-ounce steak rather than an eight-ounce steak results in a 25% reduction in calories and you probably won't notice the difference. The same can be said for all portion sizes, especially when eating out. "Supersizing" has become an American habit. It also may be one of the reasons why obesity rates have soared. So eat until you are *full* and not until you are *stuffed.*

2. **Cook with Less Fat**. It is possible, in most cases, to moderately reduce the amounts of butter, sugar, oil and cream

called for in many recipes which can significantly reduce the caloric content. When making gravies, for example, use broth instead of cream. And always use a defatting cup.

3. **Limit Access to Snacks.** Place snack food items, other than fruits and vegetables, out of sight. This will help to reduce the amount of spontaneous consumption that can really add up to a significant calorie intake throughout the day.

4. **Begin Large Meals with Soups or Salads**. This will help to satiate the appetite and may also help to cut down on large portion sizes as well as second and third helpings. It is also a good way to increase the nutrient density of the meal.

5. **Eat More Fruits and Vegetables.** Making complex carbohydrates a regular part of meal planning AND snacking will reduce caloric intake and improve the nutrient density of the diet.

6. **Limit Consumption of Fast Foods.** It is difficult, although not impossible, to get a nutritious AND low-fat meal at a fast-food restaurant. Fast-food preparation techniques produce a final product that, in many cases, is high in saturated fat, salt and sugar. As mentioned, beware of large portion sizes!

7. **Avoid Eating Meats with High Fat Content.** Processed meats such as lunch meat, sausages, hot dogs and even bacon are high in saturated fat content. Eat only lean beef and pork and stick to white meat chicken. Fish is also a lower fat source of quality protein.

8. **Improve Food Preparation Techniques.** Eat whole and or minimally cooked vegetables whenever possible. Choose baking or broiling over frying whenever you can.

9. **Variety is the Spice of Life.** And it's the same way with eating plans and diets. Not only does variety add excitement to an eating plan, it will help to assure that all of the essential nutrients from the major food groups are represented. (See The Food Guide Pyramid.)

10. **Drink Lots of Fluids.** Drinking lots of water is one of the

best ways to satiate the appetite as well as assist in the assimilation and/or digestion of all of the other nutrients. On average, about two quarts of water or fluids per day is recommended. More may be required depending upon activity level and environmental conditions.

FREQUENTLY ASKED QUESTIONS

What is a balanced diet?

A balanced diet is an eating plan that provides all of the nutrients that one needs to promote tissue growth (in other words, assists in allowing our bodies to recover from our daily tasks and/or workouts) and also provides adequate energy to meet and not exceed our daily requirement of calories. For this reason, an individual's diet or eating plan may contain more than enough calories but still might not contain enough nutrients to allow the body to perform optimally.

This is also why variety in the diet is one of the keys to balance. By choosing foods from all of the categories or groups shown in the Food Guide Pyramid and by consuming those foods in the quantities that are suggested, it is possible to modify any diet that is thought to be insufficient in terms of all of the necessary nutrients or too "rich" in certain types of foods or food groups—especially foods and food groups that contain higher amounts of saturated fats. Comparing one's actual food intake to The Food Guide Pyramid is a simple way to fine tune the diet for improved health, performance and weight management.

For example, the average American derives about 60% of his or her calories from fat and processed sugar. This is, to say the least, an imbalance that can and will have negative effects upon general health not to mention the ability to become fit through exercise. Since a large proportion of these unwanted calories are a result of heavily processed foods, it is an imbalance that can be easily overcome by tracking and analyzing one's own eating plan and making some generally minor, albeit important, adjustments.

How many calories do you need?

The number of calories that one needs to consume is dependent upon their lifestyle, activity level and weight-management goals. The body does require a certain number of calories every day in order to simply maintain what is known as "homeostasis", a state of stability or balance. In this state, the body is maintained at a healthy level and additional body weight is either gained or lost depending upon the demands placed upon it. One of the best ways to determine the number of calories that one needs each day is to calculate the "resting metabolic rate"or RMR.

The first step in determining your RMR is to calculate your body composition. As noted earlier in the book, your total body weight is a combination of your fat weight plus your lean-body mass or lean-body tissue. A certified personal trainer or fitness specialist can help you to determine these numbers by taking a few simple measurements. More information on this process will be discussed and presented in Chapter Five.

Let's assume that a 150-pound individual is found to be 20% body fat and, therefore, 80% lean-body mass (LBM). This means that the individual carries 30 pounds of fat weight (150 x .20 = 30). By subtracting the body fat weight from the total body weight, it is determined that the individual has 120 pounds of LBM (150 - 30 = 120). This number must next be converted to kilograms. By dividing the number of pounds of LBM by 2.2 we arrive at the amount of LBM in kilograms. This number is 54.55 kilograms of LBM (120/ 2.2 = 54.55). We're almost there so hang on!

Now the RMR can be determined by placing the amount of LBM measured in kilograms into the following formula: RMR = 370 + (21.6 x LBM). Now let's solve the equation.

RMR = 370 + (21.6 x 54.55)
RMR = 370 + 1178
RMR = 1548 calories

Therefore, in this example, the number of calories that the body needs IF IT REMAINS AT REST is 1548 per day. But the body doesn't remain at rest all day, although it seems that some people can do this quite well. Seriously though, this derived number must be multiplied by an activity component that estimates or approximates one's level of daily activity. If you are sedentary and participate in very little activity each day, you can multiply your RMR by 1.4. If you are moderately active and work out two or three times per week, you can multiply your

Resting Metabolic Rate (RMR) Multipliers		
Sedentary	1.4	1548 x 1.4 = 2167 calories per day
Moderately Active	1.6	1548 x 1.6 = 2477 calories per day
Extremely Active	1.8	1548 x 1.8 = 2786 calories per day

Table 4.2: Examples of Resting Metabolic Rate (RMR) for Different Activity Levels

RMR by 1.6. And if you are extremely physically active or have a job that requires lots of physical activity and, in addition, you work out three or four times per week, you should multiply your RMR by 1.8. Competitive athletes, particularly those involved in endurance sports training and competition may require even more calories. A simple review of the RMR Multipliers is listed in Table 4.2 with the total calories from the previous example included.

Are supplements necessary?

In the presence of a well-balanced diet, supplements are considered unnecessary. But how many people truly eat a balanced diet all of the time? Experts continue to suggest that supplements can help meet the Recommend Dietary Allowance (RDA) for vitamins and minerals and, in some cases, even proteins and carbohydrates. It is ALWAYS best to attempt to consume the RDA's for all of the major nutrients through a well-balanced eating plan, but there are some groups or specific populations who have been identified as being able to benefit from supplementation. These groups include:

1. Those who restrict their intake of food and, therefore, nutrients.
2. Strict vegetarians (i.e. vegetarians who eat no animal products at all).
3. Competitive athletes or athletes in training.
4. The elderly and others who may not get adequate nutrition due to their inability to eat, digest or assimilate certain foods or who may have a depressed appetite.

5. Pregnant or lactating females.
6. Individuals that take medications that may interfere with their ability to digest or assimilate certain foods or nutrients.

As can be concluded, this list can include a significant portion of the population. And as stated earlier, since we don't always eat the right kinds of foods, either by omission or commission, it does seem practical in some cases to consider dietary supplementation to ensure that we get the nutrients that may be missing from the diet. It is also a good idea for those individuals listed previous to consult a registered dietitian for more specific advise and counseling. For example, an athlete involved in rigorous training, especially strength training, may have up to twice the protein needs of a sedentary individual. If the protein does not come from the diet, it must come from somewhere and, therefore, some protein supplementation may be warranted. The special calcium and iron needs of females is another example of how supplementation may be the answer to a specific nutritional need.

In the case of vitamin and mineral supplementation, it is important that the individual be cautious so as not to exceed the RDA. This is especially true for the fat-soluble vitamins (A, D, E and K) as well as some minerals. Appendix H provides a list of the RDA's for all vitamins and selected minerals. Again, check with a registered dietitian for case-specific information on supplementation.

Are protein and amino-acid supplements necessary?

As stated earlier, a well-balanced eating plan that involves a variety of foods and follows the suggested servings in the Food Guide Pyramid will probably supply all of the amino acids (the building blocks of protein) and, therefore, protein that the body needs. With a recommended 0.8 grams of protein per kilogram of body weight (that 's 0.36 grams per POUND of body weight), it is likely that the typical diet can accommodate this amount. Indeed, as was mentioned earlier in this chapter, the American diet is very rich in protein. However, for those individuals who exercise regularly, are physically active and include strength training as a regular part of their fitness routine, additional protein

MAY be necessary. For example, it may be necessary for an individual with a comparatively higher level of lean-body mass or muscle tissue to require somewhat higher daily levels of proteins, particularly those proteins that contain the nine essential amino acids that the body cannot produce.

The foods that contain these essential amino acids are known as complete proteins and are readily available in lean meats, poultry and fish. Plant foods, such as beans, nuts, green vegetables and some starches, can also provide these nutrients but since these foods are deficient in at least one or more of the essential amino acids, they are known as incomplete proteins. This simply means that a greater variety of these types of foods are necessary to ensure an adequate supply of essential amino acids in the diet. Plant foods also are an important source of fiber in the diet and, therefore, have many other health-related benefits. Therefore, the diet or eating plan should be the first source for these nutrients before supplementation is considered. It should be noted that the National Research Council has suggested that daily intake of protein not exceed 1.6 grams per kilogram of body weight (or about 0.73 grams per pound of body weight) due to possible negative effects on the liver and kidneys. Individuals with diabetes are particularly vulnerable to these effects.

The bottom line is to analyze your eating plan carefully, or better yet have an analysis done by a registered dietitian, and supplement only when necessary and prudent with regard to specific dietary intake. By obtaining the necessary amount of protein from the regular diet, it is also more likely that the individual will be taking in more of the essential vitamins and minerals that will further enhance fitness performance and general health.

As one can see, with an honest comparison to the Food Guide Pyramid and a little bit of planning, it is possible to create an eating plan that is easy to follow and easy to make a part of one's lifestyle. And if you're blissfully happy only when eating a chocolate donut, indulge yourself every once in a while but do so in moderation and don't lose sight of the long-term goal—a fitter and healthier body.

Chapter Five
Understanding Body Composition

Most individuals who attempt a weight management program that involves either losing weight or gaining weight generally use the bathroom scale as a measure of their success or failure. But using only scale weight can be misleading and, in some cases, can actually lead to failure because of a lack of emphasis on body COMPOSITION! As discussed earlier in the book, total body weight is comprised of both fat weight and lean-body mass (LBM). It is understanding and measuring each component of total body weight individually that can help to improve both the content of the fitness program (exercise choice and diet) as well as the ability to adhere or "stick with" a fitness or weight management program in the first place.

So it's not just weight loss (or gain) that is the real program goal but, rather, an accurate assessment of and change in the total composition of the body that will allow one to successfully determine if progress is being made and/or goals are being achieved. As an example, let's assume that an individual who is starting or restarting a fitness and weight management program is 150 pounds. The goal of the program is to lose 20 pounds. In Chapter Two it was shown that a weight loss of more than about 2 to 2½ pounds per week is likely to result in a regaining of the lost weight over time. Therefore, it would be logical to assume that this weight loss could reasonably and safely occur over a period of 8 to 10 weeks. But there is a possible flaw in this scenario.

Any comprehensive weight management program that includes regular exercise (and they ALL should include regular exercise) should include strength training as a critical component. And the result of any effective strength training program will be a GAIN in LBM to at least some degree depending upon several factors such as gender (women will gain less muscle mass than men) and genetics (some individuals gain muscle mass more quickly and easily than others). It is possible, then, that one could lose 10 pounds of fat during a four-week period while gaining three pounds of lean body mass as a result of the strength training component of their program for a total weight loss of just seven pounds instead of 10 pounds. But from a body-composition standpoint this is actually a 13-pound change. The body is now leaner and the LBM component will be the real secret to PERMANENT fat loss. An understanding of "metabolic rate" will show why this is such an exciting and important concept.

The metabolic rate is the rate at which one burns calories. Nearly three-quarters of the number of calories that we burn each day is largely determined by the amount of LBM (and, more specifically, muscle mass) that we have. In fact, over 25% of the calories that we burn while we sleep is due to the caloric needs of our muscle tissue. As we age or as we become less active (or both), the body has a tendency to lose this muscle mass and/or lean tissue at a rate of about .5% to 1% each year. That's about 5 to 10 pounds of muscle loss per decade in a non-exercising adult. Each pound of muscle is lost at a metabolic cost. This means that the body is likely to be burning off less calories per day than it did a few years earlier if exercise, and particularly strength training, is not a regular part of one's lifestyle. Each pound of muscle burns a minimum of 10 to 20 calories per day. For those individuals with a higher metabolic rate, the average caloric "burn" per pound of LBM may be even higher. And the more active that a muscle is kept through exercise, the more calories are used. If food is the fuel of the body, then muscle tissue is the engine that burns it.

This is why the measurement of the amount of LBM that one has is even more important than knowing the total body weight. Weight loss (if that is the goal) is a good thing if, and only if, it does not result in a loss of lean tissue. Most "diet-only" weight-loss programs are unsuccessful because they do not address the maintenance of LBM. Also, since most "diet-only" weight-loss programs are simply low-calorie diets in disguise, it is likely that the nutrients necessary to maintain or promote muscle-tissue growth are not present in sufficient quantities. This can result in an even greater loss of muscle tissue and, therefore, an even LOWER metabolic rate. With calories being burned off at an even lower rate than before, the diet and the weight-loss program will ultimately fail.

Most successful weight-loss programs are simply a matter of regaining the muscle tissue that has been lost due to inactivity or nutrient poor diets. It is a simple process of body composition reversal, so to speak. The more LBM that is regained, the higher the natural metabolic rate (the rate at which one burns calories) is raised. The higher the natural metabolic rate is raised, the more calories that are burned ALL THE TIME—EVERY DAY—FOR-EVER!

Let's go back to our example of the 150-pound individual who wished to lose 10 pounds. As you recall, the 10-pound fat loss coupled with the three-pound LBM gain resulted in a seven-pound TOTAL weight loss rather than the desired 10 pounds after 1 month. But here's the good part: The individual is now LEANER. A smaller percentage of the individual's body is now composed of fat weight and a higher percentage is composed of lean calorie-burning tissue.

For example, if our 150-pounder was found to be 20% fat, this would mean that 30 pounds of his or her 150 pounds was composed of "adipose tissue" or fat weight and that 120 pounds was LBM. With a 10-pound fat loss coupled with the three-pound LBM gain, the current weight is now shown to be 143 pounds of total body weight. But the even better news is that total FAT weight is now only 20 pounds (about 14%) and the TOTAL LBM is now 123 pounds (about 86%). And the additional three pounds of lean body mass that was gained will produce an additional fat loss of three pounds per year as long as it is maintained with a regular routine of strength training.

Every pound of fat, whether it's on the body or in the diet, consists of 3,500 calories. As the previous example illustrates, every pound of LBM that is gained or, in most cases, REgained results in a minimum of one pound of fat loss per year. For those with slightly or even markedly higher metabolic rates, the results can be even greater! This is also why it was indicated in Chapter Four that diets alone simply don't work. They only address the amount of calories going into the body and do little to address how those calories are burned. Therefore, body composition analysis is the best and most accurate way to determine the effectiveness of any fitness and weight management program. Let's take a look at how it works.

BODY COMPOSITION ASSESSMENT TECHNIQUES AND OPTIONS

There are a number of ways to assess body composition. Let's look at several of the most common ones.

Hydrostatic Weighing

The "gold standard" for assessing body composition is hydrostatic (or underwater) weighing. It is based on the simple premise that fat floats. The individual being tested (clothed only in a bathing suit) is entirely immersed in a tank of water by being placed in a "sling" or "chair" and lowered into the tank. The nose is pinched shut using a simple nose clip and the individual being tested is asked to exhale forcefully while under the water in order to eliminate any air in the lungs. Since the "sling" is attached to a weight scale, the weight taken while the test subject is under the water is compared with the normal body weight. This determines body density and, therefore, body fat percentage can be calculated. As might be expected, this method can be expensive, time consuming and impractical due to the equipment necessary to complete the process. However, virtually all of the other methods for body composition testing are based on or compared to data collected in this manner. Clearly, hydrostatic weighing must be done in a performance laboratory setting by qualified and trained professionals. It is currently considered the most accurate method.

Skinfold Body-Composition Assessment

One of the most commonly used body-composition assessment tools is known as the skinfold method. In this method, thickness of skinfolds at specific and standardized sites on the body are taken by using a skinfold caliper (a simple device that gently squeezes the skinfolds together and indicates the thickness of the fold in millimeters). The results of all of the skinfolds are added together and placed in a formula or, more commonly, a chart that indicates percent fat. These formulas and charts are based, as stated, on the more accurate hydrostatic-weighing technique and, therefore, are considered nearly as accurate. The number of measurements taken can be as few as two or as many as a dozen or more. The standard number of measurement sites is three (although the sites for males and females differ slightly) and the measurements should always be taken by a trained and certified professional. Most commercial and private fitness centers offer this service for free or at a nominal cost. Self-assessment of skinfolds, for purposes of accuracy, is not recommended. Skinfold body-composition assessment is a simple and quick way to determine changes in body composition and should be considered a frequent (every few weeks) and regular part of the fitness program. Percent body-fat measurements my be recorded in Appendix C.

Girth Measurements

It is possible to use girth measurements as a means of determining body composition. However, it must be understood that an increase or decrease in girth measurements does not indicate which type of body tissue (fat or lean) has been increased or decreased. For this reason, it is always a good idea to supplement the information gleaned from girth measurements with body-composition analysis by other means. Measurements should be taken with a cloth or fiberglass tape to avoid inaccuracies due to stretching the tape and care should be taken to measure precisely at the same site each time. Common areas of measurement are the chest, waist, hips, thigh, calf, ankle, upper arm and wrist. Selected girth measurements may be recorded in Appendix C.

Electrical Impedance

Also known as bioelectrical impedance, this method is based upon the premise that an electrical impulse travels with less obstruction (or impedance) through lean tissue than through fatty tissue. The current used in bioelectrical-impedance testing is safe and generally imperceptible to the subject being tested. Again, it should be administered only by a trained professional. There are some challenges associated with this method that can affect its accuracy. For example, the subject might not be properly hydrated, particularly if the test is completed following a workout or even a brief bout of exercise, and it may overestimate fat deposition for some individuals with higher-than-average levels of fat-free weight and lower-than-average levels of fat weight. It is, however, relatively quick to complete. Currently, there are several easy-to-use "home" models available in a wide range of prices.

The Body-Mass Index

The Body-Mass Index or BMI is a simple estimate of body composition that simply uses height and weight. The information is plugged into a formula that is easy (trust me) to do but does require converting height from inches to meters and body weight from pounds to kilograms. The formula is: BMI = weight (kg) ÷ height squared (in meters).

Let's try an example. The subject is 5'9" and weighs 180 pounds.

First, multiply the height in inches (69 inches in this case) by 0.0254 to obtain the height in meters. [69 x 0.0254= 1.75 meters.] This number will be squared (or multiplied times itself). [1.75 x 1.75 = 3.06.]

Second, convert the weight from pounds to kilograms by dividing it by 2.2. Therefore, 180 ÷ 2.2 = 81.82 kilograms.

Now, divide the weight in kilograms by the height in meters squared. This means a BMI of 26.74. [81.82 ÷ 3.06 = 26.74.]

Based on the information in the BMI Reference Chart in Table 5.1, this indicates that this individual is considered to be in the overweight range.

A chart has also been provided in Appendix G to assist in determining this important body-composition calculation. It should be noted that body-fat percentage may also be an impor-

Weight Category	BMI Range
Normal Weight	19 to <25
Overweight	25 to <30
Obese	30 to <35
Seriously Obese	≥35

Table 5.1: BMI Reference Chart

tant factor in determining if the BMI is indicative of problems concerning overweight or obesity. This is because it is possible for an individual to have a high total body weight and a low level of fat weight and still be considered in the overweight category and, in some extreme cases, in the obese category. Although the 180-pound individual described in the earlier example may be considered overweight from the standpoint of the BMI calculation, it is possible that his fat-weight percentage may be comparatively low. This is why it is always a good idea to use more than one body-composition assessment method in determining healthy and unhealthy levels of body weight.

Waist-to-Hip Ratio

The most common type of obesity that is associated with higher levels of health risks such as heart attack and stroke is upper body obesity. This means that the predominant amounts of body fat are found above the waist and forms what has become known as the "apple" shape. To determine if this type of fat or adipose tissue distribution exists, a simple assessment known as the waist-to-hip ratio test can be easily completed and calculated. A simple measuring tape is all that is needed to make the measurements. The measurement sites are the waist at the belly button and the widest measurement of the hips or buttocks. Once the measurements are taken, the waist measurement is divided by the hip measurement to determine the ratio. For men, a hip-to-waist ratio greater than 1.0 is considered high risk and a ratio of 0.90 to 1.0 is considered a moderately high risk. For women, a waist-to-hip ratio greater than 0.85 is considered high risk while a ratio of 0.80 to 0.85 is considered a moderately high risk.

As can be easily seen, there are a variety of ways to measure body composition. Most body-composition measurements should be done every few weeks so that fitness program modifications can be made if deemed appropriate. Realizing and working toward changes in body *composition* and not just body *weight* is the optimal way to ensure progress and to be certain that the body weight being gained is LBM and that the body weight being lost is fat. As stated earlier, LBM is the real secret to permanent fat loss and successful weight management. By combining strength training with moderate levels of cardiovascular training and an eating plan that one can live with, being fit, getting fit and staying fit is easier than ever. So don't just lose *weight*, lose *fat*! There IS a difference.

Frequently Asked Questions

How much body fat is considered too much?

Acceptable "ranges" for total body-fat percentages are just that—ranges. And the factors that determine what is best for each individual also vary. Factors that are involved in controlling fat stores in the body are essentially hormonally generated but these same hormonal factors are also influenced greatly by activity or exercise levels. It is possible, therefore, for an individual to be in a range that indicates an overweight condition and still be comparatively healthy. This is why it is important to consider all of the aspects of the individual's health and fitness such as blood pressure, resting heart rate, cholesterol levels, lung function and other pertinent data in order to determine if an overweight condition is also an "overfat" condition. A simple body-composition test such as a skin-fold test can easily and quickly assess the percent-fat levels. Table 5.2 provides some guidelines for what is considered acceptable levels for adults. It must be understood that all of the levels listed are approximate and average values and, for reasons stated earlier, may not apply precisely. Lower fat levels particularly may be difficult to maintain long-term and generally are considered accurate for athletic populations and/or competitive athletes.

Also remember that these body-fat percentages will increase slightly with age at a rate of about one or two percent of fat per decade after the age of thirty.

Category	Women (% fat)	Men (% fat)
Essential fat	10-13%	2-5%
Athletes	14-20%	6-13%
Fitness	21-24%	14-17%
Healthy	25-31%	18-24%
Obese	32% and higher	25% and higher
Adapted from *Nutrition for Fitness and Sport*, 4th edition, by Melvin Williams, Brown and Benchmark Publishers.		

Table 5.2: General Body-Fat Percentage Ranges

It should also be understood that there are some individuals that are so significantly overfat (35% body fat or more) that they may have tremendous difficulty reducing their body fat to even "acceptable" levels due to a variety of factors. These individuals should realize that even a 10% loss of body fat can have significant, positive effects on the reduction of the incidence of chronic diseases and, therefore, upon their general health. This is not to say that reducing body fat to "acceptable" levels is not possible for this population but it does indicate that short-term goal setting (see Chapter Two) is important to their success and motivation.

Are there other elements of lean-body mass other than just muscle mass that can or will be increased with cardiovascular exercise and strength training?

Yes! Other than the growth of more muscle, which promotes an increase in metabolic rate (and, therefore, burns more calories), there are other lean-body mass improvements that occur. For example, since the muscle is capable of retaining more glucose (the primary source of energy for daily activities and exercise) as a result of improved fitness through exercise, more water is retained which adds to body weight. An increase in protein synthesis (muscle growth) also results in greater water volume. It is considered essential water and, therefore, does not cause bloating.

An increase in actual blood volume also occurs. Although blood does contain small amounts of lipids or fats, increased blood volume should be considered a positive effect since it means that the body can now carry more oxygen to the cells for the production of energy. Improved bone density as well as an improved density of the connective tissues (such as ligaments and tendons) will also increase lean-body mass.

Will an essential fitness program component such as strength training cause women to gain muscle at the same rate as men?

Most women are horrified at the prospect of GAINING any body weight AT ALL. They erroneously feel that they will become muscular rather than "toned" (a rather inaccurate and difficult term to define) and, therefore, will not "lose weight" while they forget that they don't want to just "lose weight," they want to lose fat! As was noted earlier, an individual's metabolic rate (the rate at which they burn calories) is predominantly determined by the amount of lean-muscle tissue that they possess as well as the oxygen-consuming capacity of that same tissue.

Secondarily, females, on average, have approximately 5 % of the typical amount of testosterone (the hormone that promotes muscle-tissue growth) that a male has and, therefore, muscular growth similar to that of a male is not possible. Some amount of muscle-tissue growth will occur but this should be considered a positive factor in that the additional amount of lean tissue that is gained will allow the individual to burn more calories PERMANENTLY—even while at rest. Over time, this will reduce the level of subcutaneous fat (the fat under the skin) as well as organic fat (fat that accumulates around the internal organs) and a leaner and more supple body will be the ultimate result. And isn't that the goal for most women?

Why do some individuals seem to have an easier time gaining or losing weight than others?

All things being equal (such as diet, regular exercise and a comprehensive fitness program), it does seem that some people do have a somewhat easier time than others in either gaining lean weight, if desired, or, more commonly, losing fat weight. We all know or have heard of those lucky folks who exercise little and eat excessively and still seem to remain "in shape" or, at least, exhibit desirable body proportions. Some seem to gain muscle mass much more easily than others and, perhaps for this reason, seem to have little trouble remaining leaner than the general population. Although these types of individuals are rare, it is frustrating at times when the rest of the "average" population must be more disciplined and adhere more strictly to a healthy eating plan and a regular exercise program.

For the most part, the reason for this disparity lies in genetics and, more succinctly, in body type or what is more correctly referred to as somatotype. There are three basic body types or somatotypes and the characteristics of one or more are observable in varying combinations in each one of us. The three body types for both males and females are known as ectomorphs , mesomorphs and endomorphs. (See Figure 5.1.) Each type has a tendency to exhibit certain characteristics in terms of body shape and structure and, as stated, many individuals exhibit some characteristics of one or more somatotypes.

The ectomorph is an individual who is genetically predisposed to lower-than-normal levels of stored body fat. They also have a somewhat more difficult time gaining lean-body mass or muscle tissue and, generally, are comparatively underweight. This does not mean that they cannot gain muscle tissue or, particularly as they age, that they cannot gain unwanted pounds in the form of fat. But it does mean that their response to different types of exercise will be...well, different and not as dramatic or marked.

The mesomorph is an individual who exhibits a tendency toward a lower or, perhaps, average level of body fat while demonstrating a marked tendency toward the gaining of lean-body mass (i.e., muscle tissue). It should be noted, however, that this

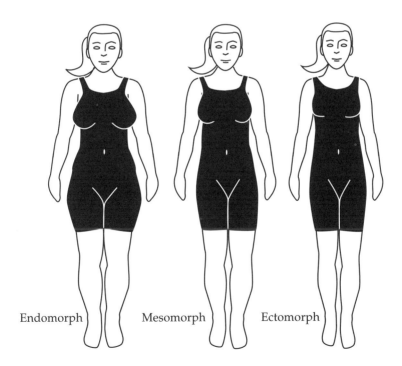

Endomorph   Mesomorph   Ectomorph

Figure 5.1: The Three Basic Body Types

body type also has a tendency to be overweight and, depending upon his or her genetics, could also gain fat weight somewhat easily, especially as the aging process progresses. With narrower hips and a comparatively wider shoulder structure, they appear to be more heavily muscled (especially males) and seem to have a more "desirable" body configuration in terms of the way the musculature develops and is naturally exhibited. For those who wish to be slender or thin, this is a body type that could have some difficulty reaching such a goal.

The third type is the endomorph. This body type exhibits a tendency toward higher levels of body fat as well as a generally higher potential for lean-body mass gain as well. A larger bone structure coupled, possibly, with a slightly lower metabolic rate would indicate that this body type would need be as consistent as possible in terms of adherence to a regular fitness program. By emphasizing the improved potential for lean-body-mass gain, following a sensible and balanced eating plan and participating in regularly scheduled cardiovascular exercise, significant fat-weight gain can be avoided and desired body shape can be maintained or achieved.

As mentioned, virtually all individuals exhibit some characteristics of one or more body types. An ectomorphic mesomorph, for example, might be characterized as exhibiting a somewhat slender yet somewhat well-muscled or "toned" body. A mesomorphic endomorph might demonstrate a positive tendency toward gaining or easily maintaining existing muscle tissue yet would need to be cognizant of their comparative greater tendency to gain fat weight. Remember that everybody is different and, therefore, EVERY BODY is different. When comparing body-composition changes or improvements, the only person who one should use for comparison is oneself. Any other comparison might, in many ways, be unfair and counterproductive due to the many genetic factors involved. Every person possesses genetic gifts and genetic burdens. The key to success is how we accept and deal with each of them. There is also, therefore, no question that, regardless of one's own particular genetic make-up, every person can improve and become more fit.

Chapter Six

Getting Started: Putting it All Together

T wo of the more difficult components to put together in any fitness program are the strength training and cardiovascular components. Generally, the reason for this challenge is, as noted, a perceived lack of time and knowing where to start or how to start. With the basic tenet that, "Any exercise is good exercise" this chapter will attempt to bring together a "starter" or "Core Program" for strength training as well as a list of activities for cardiovascular training. Using the training logs for each of the programs will also be included in the program description. Finally, a "Weekly Fitness Score" Program will be provided to bring together all of the necessary components of a comprehensive fitness plan.

THE CORE PROGRAM

The Core Program consists of several areas. They are strength training, warm-up, stretching and cardiovascular training.

Strength Training

The Core Program was developed for those individuals who have not trained with resistance exercise or weights as part of their regular fitness plan. It is also designed for those individuals who may be at a point in their strength training program where progress has become slower and a "tune-up" is in order. In any case, the five principles of a properly performed exercise described in Chapter Three should be followed precisely and carefully in order to ensure measurable progress and accurate results for each strength training workout. The reusable strength training workout card in Appendix J should be used to measure progress on a workout-by-workout basis. (This chart can be downloaded as a full 8½ x 11 page at www.cardinalpub.com/befit.)

The exercises/lifts suggested on the strength training workout card should be accomplished, whenever possible, in the order suggested. The number of exercises/lifts for each body part is also suggested right on the card. Simply date the card for each workout and, next to each exercise/lift accomplished with proper form, record the number of repetitions completed below the slanted line and the amount of weight or resistance used above the slanted line as shown in Chapter Three. Remember, only record the number of repetitions completed WITHIN THE SPECIFIED REPETITION RANGE on the FIRST set of exercise.

To establish a "base" or beginning level as described in Chapter Three, remember that, for the upper body, the ability to complete more than 12 repetitions means that the weight is probably too light and the inability to complete at least 8 repetitions means that the weight is too heavy. For the lower body, the suggested range is 10 to 15 repetitions. Once the base level has been established (and it may take two or three workouts to accomplish this), it is suggested that only one set of exercise be completed at each workout for the first two to four weeks. For more experienced exercisers, one to three sets is suggested using the Quick Set System described in detail in Chapter Three.

The workout card shown in Appendix J will list many different exercises for the various parts of the body. Only those exercises marked with an asterisk (*) are part of The Core Program. Additional lifts or exercises are listed to allow for eventual program expansion and to add variety to the existing program.

Core Program Summary

I.   Warm-up
II. Stretching
III. Lower Body
    a. Leg Extension
    b. Leg Curl (front lying or seated)
    c. Leg Press
IV. Upper Body
    a. Chest Press (machine, barbell or dumbbell)
    b. Seated Row or Bent Row (dumbbell)
    c. Seated Press (machine or dumbbells)
    d. Curl-ups
    e. Twisting Curl-ups

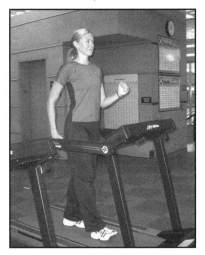 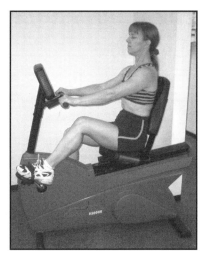

Both treadmill walking and riding an exercise bicycle are good warm-ups.

Warm-Up

Before beginning any strength training program, it is suggested that 5 to 10 minutes of light to moderate aerobic exercise be completed. This can take the form of simple calisthenics such as jumping jacks or can consist of brisk walking or use of a stationary bike. A light sweat is a good indication that the body is now warmed-up sufficiently for exercise.

Stretching

A few minutes of stretching the major muscle groups of the body (see Chapter 1) is suggested before beginning the strength workout. It should be remembered that stretching problem areas such as the low back and hamstrings are recommended just before and just after the specific body parts are trained with resistance exercise.

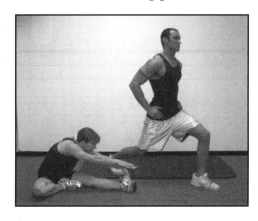

THE CORE PROGRAM

Lower Body

Leg Extension: works quadricep muscles (front of thigh)

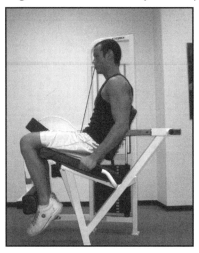 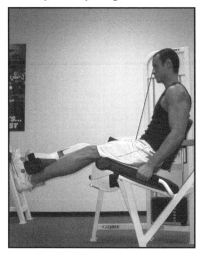

As Shown:

- Adjust the seat so that the knee joints are aligned with the axis of rotation.
- Stabilize by using the handgrips.
- Position the ankles behind the movement pad.
- Raise the lever arm in about 1-2 seconds by extending the legs.
- Pause momentarily in the full contracted position.
- Return to the starting position in about 3-4 seconds and repeat.

Beginner
Number of Sets: 1   Repetition Range: 10-15

Experienced
Number of Sets: 1-3   Repetition Range: 10-15

THE CORE PROGRAM

Lower Body

Leg Curl (prone): works hamstring muscles (back of thigh)

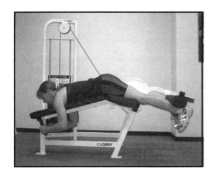 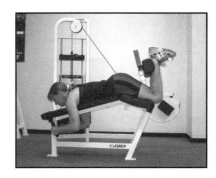

As Shown:
- Lie face down on the pads of the machine
- Stabilize by using the handgrips.
- Place the ankles under the pad.
- Align the knees with the axis of rotation.
- Raise the lever arm in about 1-2 seconds by flexing the legs.
- Pause momentarily in full contracted position.
- Return to the starting position in about 3-4 seconds and repeat.

Beginner
Number of Sets: 1   Repetition Range: 10-15

Experienced
Number of Sets: 1-3   Repetition Range: 10-15

THE CORE PROGRAM

Lower Body

Leg Curl (seated): works hamstring muscles (back of thigh)

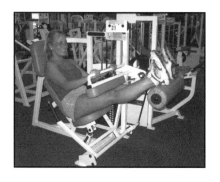 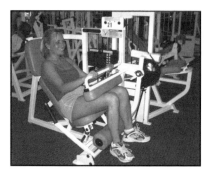

As Shown:

- Adjust seat so that the knee joints are aligned with the axis of rotation.
- Extend the legs and place backs of the ankles on top of the lever pad.
- Adjust and position the thigh stabilizer pad on top of the thigh.
- Pull the lever arm down in about 1-2 seconds by flexing the legs.
- Pause momentarily in the full contracted position.
- Return to the starting position in about 3-4 seconds and repeat.

Beginner
Number of Sets: 1   Repetition Range: 10-15

Experienced
Number of Sets: 1-3 Repetition Range: 10-15

THE CORE PROGRAM

Lower Body

Leg Press: works hips and legs

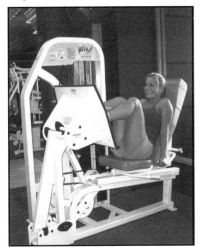 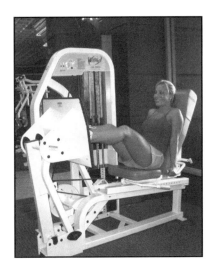

As Shown:

- Sit on the seat with the feet placed evenly on the foot platform.
- Stabilize by using the handgrips.
- Push the foot platform forward in about 1-2 seconds by extending the legs and hips.
- Do not completely lock out at the knee joint.
- Pause momentarily, in the full contracted position.
- Return to the starting position in about 3-4 seconds and repeat.

Beginner
Number of Sets: 1   Repetition Range: 10-15

Experienced
Number of Sets: 1-3   Repetition Range: 10-15

THE CORE PROGRAM

Upper Body

Chest Press (machine): works pectorals (chest) and triceps (upper arm)

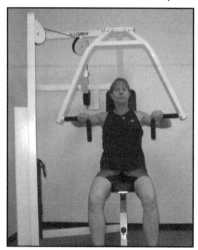 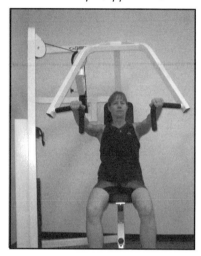

As Shown:

- Adjust the seat so that the bar grips are even with the middle of the chest.
- Place the hands on the bar grips so that the chest is in a slightly stretched position, to begin.
- Press out in about 1-2 seconds to a near lock-out position by extending the arms.
- The arms should be perpendicular to the body at the full extension.
- Pause momentarily in the full contracted position.
- Return to the starting position in about 3-4 seconds.

Beginner
Number of Sets: 1   Repetition Range: 8-12

Experienced
Number of Sets: 1-3   Repetition Range: 8-12

THE CORE PROGRAM

Upper Body

Chest Press (barbell): works pectorals (chest) and triceps (upper arm)

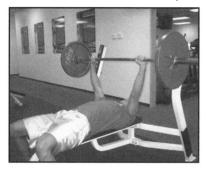 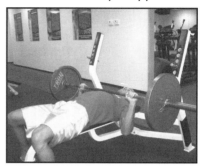

As Shown:

- Position the bar over the chest with the arms extended.
- Lower the bar using a controlled movement in about 3-4 seconds until the bar touches the chest.
- Pause momentarily in this position.
- Return to the starting position in about 1-2 seconds by extending the arms and repeat.

Beginner
Number of Sets: 1   Repetition Range: 8-12

Experienced
Number of Sets: 1-3 Repetition Range: 8-12

THE CORE PROGRAM

Upper Body

Chest Press (dumbbells): works pectorals (chest) and triceps (upper arm)

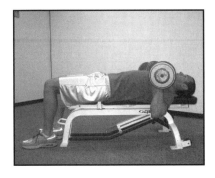 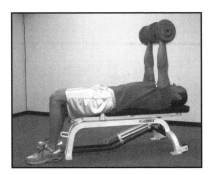

As Shown:

- Lie on the back on a padded bench.
- Position the dumbbells at chest level.
- Press the dumbbells away from the chest in about 1-2 seconds by extending the arms.
- Pause momentarily in this position.
- Lower dumbbells to the starting position in about 3-4 seconds and repeat.

Beginner
Number of Sets: 1   Repetition Range: 8-12

Experienced
Number of Sets: 1-3   Repetition Range: 8-12

THE CORE PROGRAM

Upper Body

Seated Row: works latisimus dorsi (upper back), posterior deltoid (rear shoulder) and triceps (upper arm)

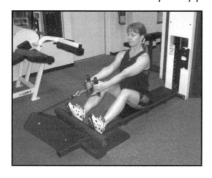 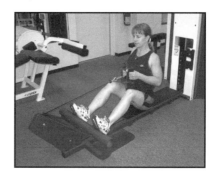

As Shown:

- From a seated position with the legs slightly bent and the back straight, grasp the resistance bar.
- With the arms straight, pull the resistance toward the upper torso in about 1-2 seconds (in a line parallel to the floor) by flexing the arms.
- Pause momentarily when the resistance bar touches or nears the chest.
- Lower the resistance to the starting position in about 3-4 seconds and repeat.

Beginner
Number of Sets: 1   Repetition Range: 8-12

Experienced
Number of Sets: 1-3   Repetition Range: 8-12

THE CORE PROGRAM

Upper Body

Bent Over Row (dumbbell): works latisimus dorsi (upper back), posterior deltoid (rear shoulder) and biceps (upper arm)

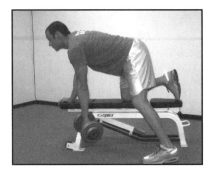 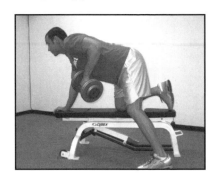

As Shown:

- Using a flat bench, position the knee and hand to support the upper body so that the torso is slightly higher than parallel to the floor.
- The supporting arm should be perpendicular to the floor to adequately support the upper body.
- Grasp the dumbbell and allow the dumbbell to hang directly down from the shoulder.
- Pull the dumbbell up to or close to the chest in about 1-2 seconds by flexing the arm.
- Pause momentarily in the fully contracted position.
- Lower the dumbbell to the starting position in about 3-4 seconds and repeat.

Beginner
Number of Sets: 1   Repetition Range: 8-12

Experienced
Number of Sets: 1-3   Repetition Range: 8-12

THE CORE PROGRAM

Upper Body

Seated Press (machine): works deltoids (shoulders) and triceps (upper arm)

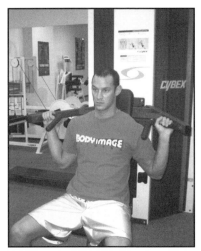 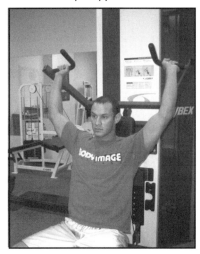

As Shown:
- Adjust the seat height so that the elbows are as low as possible at the starting position and grasp the resistance bar.
- Press the resistance bar upward in about 1-2 seconds to a near lock-out position by extending the arms.
- Pause momentarily in the full contracted position.
- Lower the resistance to the starting position in about 3-4 seconds and repeat.

Beginner
Number of Sets: 1   Repetition Range: 8-12

Experienced
Number of Sets: 1-3   Repetition Range: 8-12

THE CORE PROGRAM

Upper Body

Seated Press (dumbbell): works deltoids (shoulders) and triceps (upper arm)

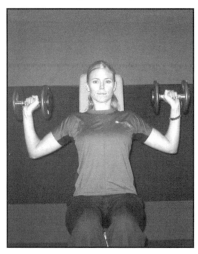 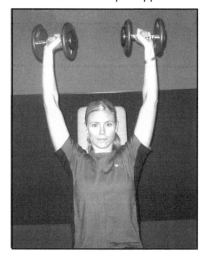

As Shown:

- Assume a seated position on a bench (preferably a bench with back support) and grasp the dumbbells.
- Position the dumbbells with the arms bent and the dumbbells at approximately the level of the shoulders.
- Press the dumbbells upward in about 1-2 seconds to a near lockout position by extending the arms.
- Pause momentarily in the full contracted position.
- Lower the dumbbells to the starting position in 3-4 seconds and repeat.

Beginner
Number of Sets: 1   Repetition Range: 8-12

Experienced
Number of Sets: 1-3   Repetition Range: 8-12

THE CORE PROGRAM

Upper Body

Curl-ups: works rectus abdominus (stomach area)

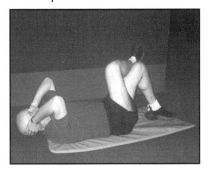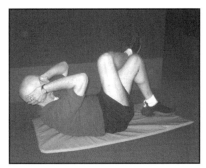

As Shown:

- Lie flat on the back on a mat or other similar surface with the knees bent and one leg crossed over the other.
- Place the hands on the side of the head with the arms bent and the elbows pointed forward. Support the head gently with the fingers.
- Curl the upper torso forward in about 1-2 seconds by attempting to bring the elbows as close to the knees of the crossed leg as possible. (Curl straight forward with no twisting movement.)
- Pause momentarily in the full contracted position.
- Lower to the starting position in about 3-4 seconds and repeat.

Beginner and Experienced

Repetition Range: 10-15, with the right leg crossed over the left leg. 10-15, with the left leg crossed over the right leg. If at least 10 repetitions cannot be accomplished, do as many as possible until the desired number is reached.

THE CORE PROGRAM

Upper Body

Twisting Curl-ups: works rectus abdominus (stomach area) and external obliques (side of stomach area)

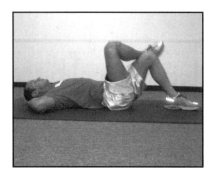 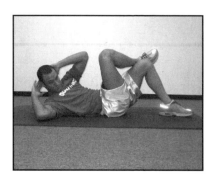

As Shown:

- Lie flat on the back on a mat or other similar surface with the knees bent and one leg crossed over the other.
- Place the hands behind the head with the elbows out to the side and touching the mat or floor. Support the head gently with the fingers.
- Curl the upper torso up and across the mid-line of the body in about 1-2 seconds by attempting to bring the left elbow to the right knee while keeping the right elbow in contact with the mat.
- Pause momentarily in the full contracted position.
- Return to the starting position in about 3-4 seconds and repeat.

Beginner and Experienced
Repetition Range: 10-15, with the right leg crossed over the left leg. 10-15, with the left leg crossed over the right leg. If at least 10 repetitions cannot be accomplished, do as many as possible until the desired number is reached.

All exercises should be completed in the prescribed order and multiple sets for experienced lifters should incorporate, where possible, the Quick Set System to reduce total training time. (See the Quick Set System in Chapter Three for review). Results from the first set of each listed exercise should be recorded on the strength training card.

The program should be completed two to three days per week with a minimum of 48 to 72 hours (two to three days) in between each workout. This will allow for sufficient training stimulus as well as sufficient and necessary recovery time. Remember to record the date of each workout. Cardiovascular training can take place on the same day as the strength training program or on alternate days depending upon one's personal schedule. It is generally considered safer to do the cardiovascular program before the strength program if both are done on the same day.

The Core Program allows the individual to train all of the major muscle groups efficiently, effectively and in an optimal order. It is for beginners or for those who wish to restart their program after a period of inactivity or due to lack of success in their current program. **Please note that the Core Program uses one exercise/lift for each muscle group.** Training of the arms is accomplished within the exercise/life choices inherent in the program. However, if additional arm training is desired, those exercises/lifts can be completed or added to the program after initial success with the Core Program has been accomplished. These additional exercises are listed on the strength training workout card in Appendix J and described on the following pages.

ADDITIONAL EXERCISES AND LIFTS

Upper Body

Bent Arm Fly (machine): works pectorals (chest) and anterior deltoid (front shoulder)

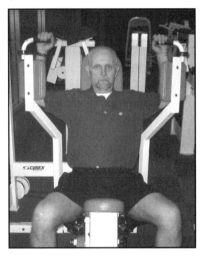 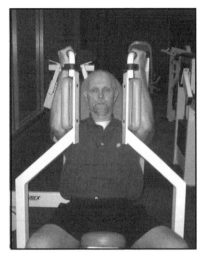

As Shown:

- Adjust the seat so that the upper arm is slightly above parallel to the floor when the forearms are placed against the resistance pads and hands are placed on the hand grips.
- Press the resistance pads forward and toward the midline of the body in about 1-2 seconds until the elbows are pointed directly forward.
- Pause momentarily in the full contracted position.
- Lower the resistance to the starting position in about 3-4 seconds and repeat.

Beginner
Number of Sets: 1   Repetition Range: 8-12

Experienced
Number of Sets: 1-3   Repetition Range: 8-12

ADDITIONAL EXERCISES AND LIFTS

Upper Body

Bent Arm Fly (dumbbell): works pectorals (chest) and anterior deltoid (front of shoulder)

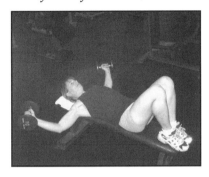 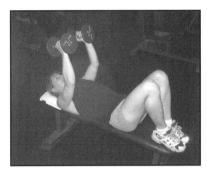

As Shown:

- Lie on the back on a padded bench.
- Grasp the dumbbells in an extended-arm position to the sides with a slight bend in the arms at the elbows and the arms perpendicular to the axis of the body.
- While maintaining the angle of the arm at the elbow (arms nearly extended), draw the dumbbells up and toward the midline of the body in about 1-2 seconds.
- Pause momentarily in the full contracted position.
- Lower the resistance to the starting position in about 3-4 seconds and repeat.

Beginner
Number of Sets: 1   Repetition Range: 8-12

Experienced
Number of Sets: 1-3   Repetition Range: 8-12

ADDITIONAL EXERCISES AND LIFTS

Upper Body

Lat Pulldown (narrow grip; preferred): works latisimus dorsi (upper back) and biceps (upper arm)

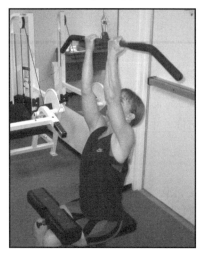 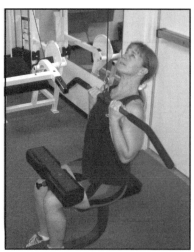

As Shown:

- Adjust the seat in the machine so that the thigh pads assist in stabilizing the lower body.
- Grasp the resistance bar using a chin-up grip (palms toward the face) with the arms shoulder-width apart and completely extended.
- Pull the resistance bar down to the chest in about 1-2 seconds by flexing the arms.
- Pause momentarily iun the full contracted position.
- Return to starting position in about 3-4 seconds and repeat.

Beginner
Number of Sets: 1   Repetition Range: 8-12

Experienced
Number of Sets: 1-3 Repetition Range: 8-12

ADDITIONAL EXERCISES AND LIFTS

Upper Body

Lat Pulldown (wide grip): works latisimus dorsi (upper back) and biceps (upper arm)

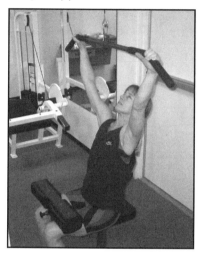 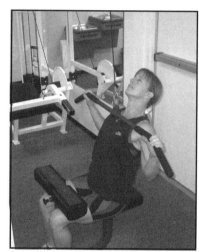

As Shown:

- Adjust the seat in the machine so that the thigh pads assist in stabilizing the lower body.
- Grasp the resistance bar using a wide grip (palms facing away from the face) with the arms slightly wider than shoulder-width apart and completely extended.
- Pull resistance bar down to the chest in about 1-2 seconds by flexing the arms.
- Pause momentarily in the full contracted position.
- Return to starting position in about 3-4 seconds and repeat.

Beginner
Number of Sets: 1   Repetition Range: 8-12

Experienced
Number of Sets: 1-3 Repetition Range: 8-12

ADDITIONAL EXERCISES AND LIFTS

Upper Body

Pullover (machine): works laisimus dorsi (upper back)

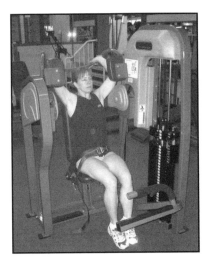 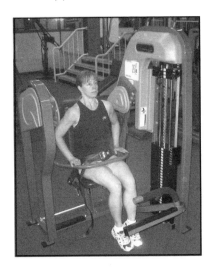

As Shown:

- Sit in the seat and adjust the seat height so that the shoulders are even with the axis of rotation of the machine.
- Fasten the seat beat to stabilize the lower body.
- Press on the foot lever to bring the movement pads into reach.
- Place the elbows on the pads and gently grasp the cross bar.
- Release the foot pedal.
- Pull the movement pads down in about 1-2 seconds until the resistance bar touches the lap or thigh.
- Pause momentarily in the full contracted position.
- Return the resistance bar to the starting position in about 3-4 seconds and repeat.

Beginner   Number of Sets: 1   Repetition Range: 8-12

Experienced Number of Sets: 1-3 Repetition Range: 8-12

ADDITIONAL EXERCISES AND LIFTS

Upper Body

Lateral Raise (machine): works deltoids (shoulders)

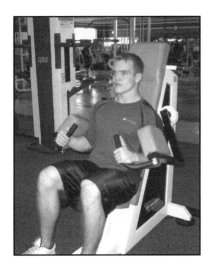 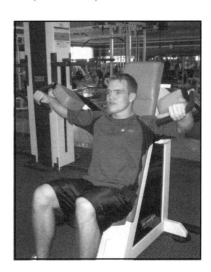

As Shown:

- Adjust the seat so that the shoulders are aligned with the axis of rotation of the machine. If available, adjust the seat belt.
- Grasp the hand grips and place the upper arms against the movement pads.
- Lift the movment pads in about 1-2 seconds until the lever arms are parallel to the floor.
- Pause momentarily in the full contracted position.
- Return to the starting position in about 3-4 seconds and repeat.

Beginner
Number of Sets: 1   Repetition Range: 8-12

Experienced
Number of Sets: 1-3   Repetition Range: 8-12

ADDITIONAL EXERCISES AND LIFTS

Upper Body

Lateral Raise (dumbbells): works deltoids (shoulders)

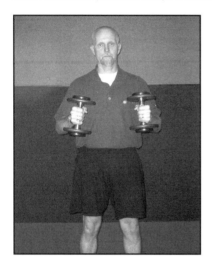 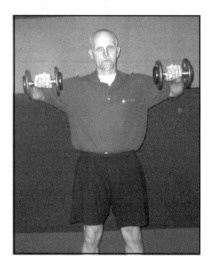

As Shown:

- Stand firmly with the feet approximately shoulder-width apart.
- Grasp the dumbbelsl and, with arms bent at about a 90-degree angle, position the dumbbells in front of the torso.
- Raise the resistance up and away from the body in about 1-2 seconds until the upper arm is parallel to the floor. (Maintain arm angle throughout.)
- Pause momentarily in the full contracted position.
- Return to the starting position in about 3-4 seconds and repeat.

Beginner
Number of Sets: 1   Repetition Range: 8-12

Experienced
Number of Sets: 1-3   Repetition Range: 8-12

ADDITIONAL EXERCISES AND LIFTS

Upper Body

Upright Row: works deltoids (shoulders) and biceps (upper arm)

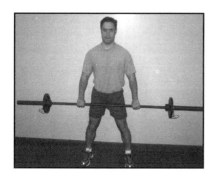 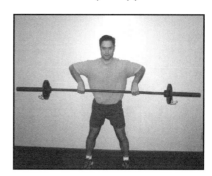

As Shown:
- Stand with the feet approximately shoulder-width apart and grasp the barbell with the hands slightly wider than the feet.
- The barbell should hang straight down at approximately hip level.
- Raise the barbell up in about 1-2 seconds until the upper arms are parallel to the floor.
- Pause momentarily in the full contracted position.
- Lower the barbell to the starting position in about 3-4 seconds and repeat.

Beginner
Number of Sets: 1   Repetition Range: 8-12

Experienced
Number of Sets: 1-3   Repetition Range: 8-12

ADDITIONAL EXERCISES AND LIFTS

Lower Body

Squat: works hips and legs

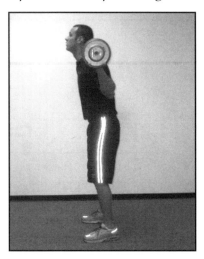 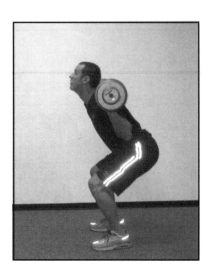

As Shown:

- Place the barbell across the upper part of the shoulders and back and grasp it firmly. (A power or squat rack is recommended for safety.)
- Position the feet slightly wider than shoulder-width apart.
- Lower the hips in about 1-2 seconds until the thighs are almost parallel to the floor.
- Pause momentarily in this position.
- Raise the hips back to the starting position in about 3-4 seconds and repeat.
- Keep the back as erect as possible throughout the exercise.
- A spotter is always recommended!

Beginner
Number of Sets: 1   Repetition Range: 15-20 (with lower weight)

Experienced
Number of Sets: 1-3   Repetition Range: 10-15

ADDITIONAL EXERCISES AND LIFTS

Lower Body

Calf Raise (seated): works gastrocnemius and soleus (calves)

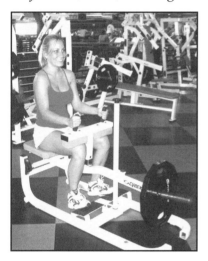 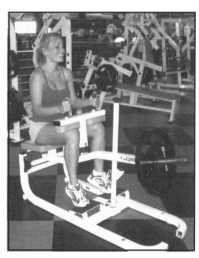

As Shown:

- Assume a seated position and adjust the thigh pads onto the tops of the thighs.
- Place the hands on the handgrips. Place the balls of the feet on the foot platform with the heels down and the backs of the ankles in the stretched position (heels below the foot platform).
- Raise the resistance in about 1-2 seconds by lifting the heels as high as possible, simulating a toe raise. Release the restraint bar.
- Pause momentarily in the full contracted position.
- Lower the resistance in about 3-4 seconds to the starting position with the heels below the foot platform and repeat. Replace the restraint bar after the positive phase of the final repetition and lower slowly to re-rack the resistance.

Beginner   Number of Sets: 1   Repetition Range: 15-20

Experienced Number of Sets: 1-3 Repetition Range: 10-15

ADDITIONAL EXERCISES AND LIFTS

Upper Body

Bicep Curl (machine): works biceps (upper arm)

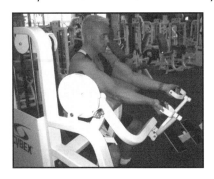 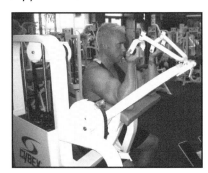

As Shown:

- Adjust the seat so that the elbow joints are aligned with the axis of rotation of the machine. (The backs of the arms should remain in contact with the pads throughout.)
- Grasp the handles with palms up.
- Lift handles up in about 1-2 seconds until the biceps are fully contracted or the handles are near the face.
- Pause momentarily in the full contracted position.
- Return the resistance to the starting position in about 3-4 seconds and repeat.

Beginner
Number of Sets: 1   Repetition Range: 8-12

Experienced
Number of Sets: 1-3   Repetition Range: 8-12

ADDITIONAL EXERCISES AND LIFTS

Upper Body

Bicep Curl (barbell): works biceps (upper arms)

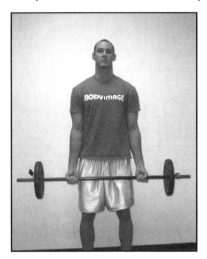 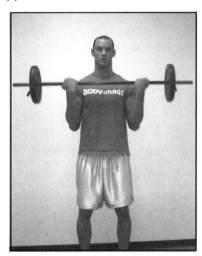

As Shown:
- Stand erect with the feet about shoulder-width apart.
- Grasp the barbell with an underhand grip, the arms extended down and the bar at the level of the hips.
- Curl the barbell upward in about 1-2 seconds until it touches or nears the chest.
- Pause momentarily in the full contracted position.
- Lower the barbell in about 3-4 seconds to the starting position and repeat.

Beginner
Number of Sets: 1   Repetition Range: 8-12

Experienced
Number of Sets: 1-3   Repetition Range: 8-12

ADDITIONAL EXERCISES AND LIFTS

Upper Body

Bicep Curl (Dumbbell): works biceps (upper arms)

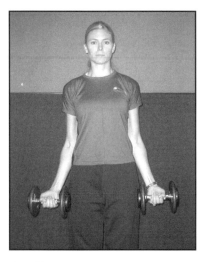 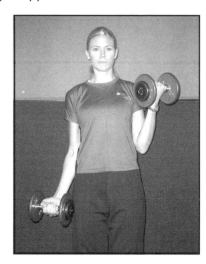

As Shown:

- Assume a standing position with the feet about shoulder-width apart.
- Grasp the dumbbells in both hands with the arms extended down and the palms facing out.
- Curl one dumbbell upward in about 1-2 seconds until it touches or nears the shoulder.
- Pause momentarily in the full contracted position.
- Lower the dumbbell in about 3-4 seconds and repeat.
- Repeat the procedure with the opposite arm.
- This exercise can also be completed by lifting both dumbbells simultaneously.

Beginner
Number of Sets: 1   Repetition Range: 8-12

Experienced
Number of Sets: 1-3   Repetition Range: 8-12

ADDITIONAL EXERCISES AND LIFTS

Upper Body

Tricep Push Down: works triceps (upper arm)

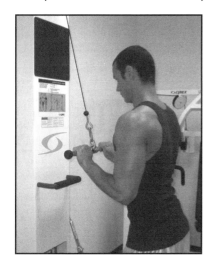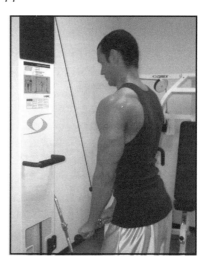

As Shown:

- Assume a standing position in front of the tricep-cable machine.
- Grasp the resistance bar in front of the tricep-cable machine with the palms down.
- Push the resistance bar down in about 1-2 seconds until both arms are completely extended.
- Pause momentarily in the full contracted position.
- Return to the starting position in about 3-4 seconds and repeat.

Beginner
Number of Sets: 1   Repetition Range: 8-12

Experienced
Number of Sets: 1-3   Repetition Range: 8-12

Cardiovascular Training

Nearly a dozen suggested cardiovascular training activities are listed for you on the Cardio Training Log (Appendix B). Refer to that card log and circle one or two activities that you enjoy or would like to try as your workout. Follow these general guidelines:

1. List the time and distance that was completed on your cardiovascular workout or activity—even if it was just a brisk walk.

2. Enter your heart rate while you were exercising. This "training heart rate" should be taken about 10 minutes into the exercise bout (not including the warm-up) and every 10 or 15 minutes thereafter. Record the highest heart rate taken during the chosen exercise or activity.

3. List any comments concerning your workout in the comment section and date the entry. This will help you to choose exercises more effectively in terms of performance and perception.

4. Periodically compare your heart-rate responses to similar exercise routines. In this way, you can determine if you are improving by checking to see if your heart-rate response to similar exercise workloads is going down. If so, you are becoming more aerobically fit; if not, you may need to modify the intensity or the duration of the exercise bouts——or even choose a new or different exercise. (See Chapter Three regarding exercise intensity.)

5. Perform your chosen activity three to five times per week for a minimum of 20 and a maximum of 60 minutes per day.

6. If you are a beginner and can only do five or ten minutes of cardiovascular exercise, use the initial time frame as a starting point and gradually add more time to your exercise routine (a minute or two per week, for example) before increasing the intensity.

7. Be patient in looking for cardiovascular improvements.

8. Cool down gradually after training.

9. Drink plenty of water both before and after training, especially if training in a hot and/or humid environment.

Consider training indoors in a climate-controlled environment on very hot and/or humid days.

10. Stretch for a few minutes after you have cooled down a bit and your training routine is completed. (See Chapter One for some suggested flexibility exercises.)

It is easy to see, then, just how simple it is to begin and to follow through with these fundamental and effective methods of training the musculoskeletal and cardiovascular systems. Establishing base levels for both strength and cardiovascular fitness—no matter how low—and beginning with moderate levels of exercise as part of a regular routine will, over time, not only show improvements in fitness levels on paper but will result in a healthier, more energetic and more fit individual. As stated earlier, there is no such thing as a bad exercise and by keeping track of some simple and easy to measure workout information, it is possible to see on a workout-by-workout basis just how much improvement is taking place.

PUTTING IT ALL TOGETHER

In order to bring together all of the components of a total fitness program, a weekly score sheet has been placed in Appendix I. Again, this score sheet, the Fitness Points Log, is detachable and can be copied over and over again to illustrate just how well your fitness program is doing and just how balanced it is. Points are assigned for different aspects of the fitness plan including strength training, cardiovascular training and eating plans. There is even a place where points are awarded for many common everyday activities that, when ACTIVELY pursued, do help to improve general fitness levels. All of the components, of course, will impact positively upon body composition and weight management. It is a fun way to determine the comprehensiveness of one's fitness program since emphasis on only one area alone (such as diet alone or cardiovascular training alone) is, generally and in the long term, a recipe for failure.

It should also be noted that there is both a daily and weekly limit on the number of points that are possible so that no one area of the fitness program is overemphasized and so that overtraining in certain areas does not take place. The Fitness Points

BE FIT, STAY FIT!

Log should be filled out weekly and the points tallied to see if the fitness program is balanced and to make sure that the main components of a comprehensive program are being addressed.

Epilogue

There is no book, instructional manual or text that can adequately cover all of the areas in "fitness" or answer all of the questions about exercise and its relationship to health. At an early stage of my professional development, I was taught by one of my advisors and mentor, Dr. Karl Stoedefalke, that man is truly a creature of movement and secretions and when the movement ceases or slows down significantly, the creature begins to become diseased. I also realized after many years as a strength and conditioning coach and personal trainer to thousands of individuals in both athletic and non-athletic populations that exercise IS medicine. But since everybody is different and, therefore, everybody has a somewhat different definition of fitness or has slightly different goals and/or potentials, it is almost impossible to explain every topic or area of fitness and its myriad components in a way that is applicable to all.

What I have attempted to do in this book is to give real-world answers and explanations to real-world questions and concerns regarding a rather wide variety of fitness issues. After being asked to respond to these questions and concerns for more than two decades, this book was written in a humble attempt to show that exercise is for everyone and that everyone can—and must—participate in regular exercise. In that attempt, I have tried to keep the explanations simple and the tone of the book instructive and conversational. I also tried to inject a little bit of humor into the mix whenever I could.

My greatest hope, however, is to motivate those individuals who are sedentary or, for whatever reason, have lost hope that exercise is a viable way to overcome many of the chronic illnesses brought about by being overweight or obese. The many benefits of a healthy and fit lifestyle are possible for EVERYONE and every investment that an individual makes in their own health is an investment that pays dividends for themselves as well as the people around them. For those who are quite active and already convinced of the benefits of a fitter and healthier body, this book has attempted to demonstrate that a regular program of fitness can be accomplished in an efficient and effective manner. After all, meaningful human movement is what we were created to do. It's in our genetic code! And if we ignore or squander the opportunity to become healthy or remain healthy through exercise and properly focused eating plans, we have really been unfaithful to ourselves as the creatures of movement that we truly are.

So don't stop learning about fitness and health. And never stop using your gift—your body—in a way that promotes fitness and wellness. No matter how much or how little exercise you do, it's all good! Enjoy the journey and keep your eye on the prize. I KNOW you can do it!

Paul M. Kennedy, Ed.D.

Appendices

Regular physical activity is fun and healthy and increasingly more people are starting to become more active every day. Being more active is very safe for most people. However, some people should check with their doctor before they can start becoming much more physically active.

If you are planning to become much more physically active than you are now, start by answering the seven questions in the box below. If you are between the ages of 15 and 69, the Par-Q will tell you if you should check with your doctor before you start. If you are over 66 years of age and you are not used to be very active, check with your doctor.

Common sense is your best guide when you answer these questions. Please read the questions carefully and answer each one honestly.

YES	NO		
☐	☐	1.	Has your doctor ever said that you have a heart condition and that you should only do physical actvity recommended by a doctor?
☐	☐	2.	Do you feel pain in your chest when you do physical activity?
☐	☐	3.	In the past month, have you had chest pain when you were not doing physical activity?
☐	☐	4.	Do you lose your balance because of dizziness or do you ever lose consciousness?
☐	☐	5.	Do you have a bone or joint problem that could be made worse by a change in your physical activity?
☐	☐	6.	Is you doctor currently prescribing drugs (for example, water pills) for your blood pressure or heart condition?
☐	☐	7.	Do you know of any other reason why you should not do physical activity?

If you answered YES to one or more questions:
- Talk with your doctor by phone or in person before you start becoming much more physically active or before you have a fitness appraisal. Tell your doctor about the PAR-Q and the questions you answered YES.
- You may be able to do any activity you want, as long as you start slowly and build up gradually. Or, you may need to restrict your activities to those which are safe for you. Talk with your doctor about the kinds of activities you wish to participate in and follow his/her advice.
- Find out which community programs are safe and healthful for you.

If you answered NO to all questions:
- If you answered No to all PAR-Q questions, you can be reasonably sure that you can start becoming much more phsyically active — begin slowly and build up gradually. This is the safest way to to. You can also take part in a fitness appraisal — this is an excellent way to determine your basic fitness so that you can plan the best way for you to live actively.

Appendix B: Cardio Training Log				
Activity/Date				
Walking *Time:*				
Distance or Workload				
Heart Rate				
Brisk Walking *Time:*				
Distance or Workload				
Heart Rate				
Running *Time:*				
Distance or Workload				
Heart Rate				
Rowing *Time:*				
Distance or Workload				
Heart Rate				
Swimming *Time:*				
Distance or Workload				
Heart Rate				
Step Machine *Time:*				
Distance or Workload				
Heart Rate				
Elliptical Trainer *Time:*				
Distance or Workload				
Heart Rate				
Stationary Bike *Time:*				
Distance or Workload				
Heart Rate				
Biking *Time:*				
Distance or Workload				
Heart Rate				
Other *Time:*				
Distance or Workload				
Heart Rate				

Note: The cardio training log can be downloaded at www.cardinalpub.com/befit

APPENDIX C: Body Composition Measurements

DATE							GOAL
WEIGHT							
% BODY FAT							
LEAN MASS							
FAT WEIGHT							

*SELECTED BODY PART MEASUREMENTS

CHEST							
WAIST							
HIP							
THIGH							
OTHER							

Fat Weight=Body Weight x Percent Body Fat   Lean Mass=Body Weight - Fat Weight

- *Chest and hips circumference measurements taken at widest point.*
- *Waist circumference measurements taken at umbilicus (belly button).*
- *Thigh circumference measurement taken midway between knee and hip joint.*

Flexibility Measurements: Sit and Reach Test

DATE	SCORE

NOTE: Body-composition and flexibility measurements should be recorded every two to four weeks or as desired.

Appendix D: Eating Plan Diary (EPD)	
DAYS/DATES:	Number of Servings
Foods consumed (description)	
BREAKFAST:	
LUNCH:	
DINNER:	
OTHER MEAL:	
ALL SNACKS:	

NOTES:

1. Record all foods that you ate during a 24-hour period

2. List the servings from the meat group in ounces.

3. **The Eating Plan Diary can be downloaded at www.cardinalpub.com/befit**

Appendix E: Eating Plan Analysis (EPA)							
		SUGGESTED SERVINGS FOR SPECIFIC CALORIC INTAKES					
FOOD GROUP	*SERVINGS*	*1,600*	*2,200*	*2,800*	*CIRCLE ONE*		
Fats Oils and Sweets		<2	<2	<2	Too Little	Adequate	Too Much
Milk, Yogurt and Cheese		2	3	3	Too Little	Adequate	Too Much
Meat, Poultry, Fish, Dried Beans, Eggs and Nuts		5	6	7	Too Little	Adequate	Too Much
Vegetable		2	3	3	Too Little	Adequate	Too Much
Fruit		2	3	4	Too Little	Adequate	Too Much
Bread, Cereal, Rice and Pasta		6	9	11	Too Little	Adequate	Too Much
Water		8	8	8	Too Little	Adequate	Too Much

NOTES:

1. *Record your intake of water in an eight-ounce servings.*

2. *List the servings from the meat group in ounces.*

3. *The Eating Plan Analysis can be downloaded at www.cardinalpub.com/befit*

Appendix F: The Food Guide Pyramid

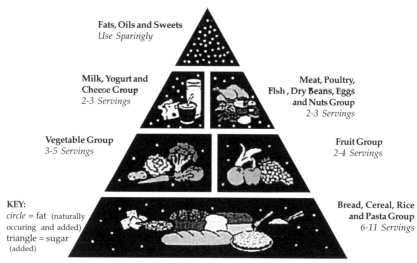

Fats, Oils and Sweets
Use Sparingly

Milk, Yogurt and Cheese Group
2-3 Servings

Meat, Poultry, Fish, Dry Beans, Eggs and Nuts Group
2-3 Servings

Vegetable Group
3-5 Servings

Fruit Group
2-4 Servings

KEY:
circle = fat (naturally occuring and added)
triangle = sugar (added)

Bread, Cereal, Rice and Pasta Group
6-11 Servings

These symbols show fats and added sugars in food

What counts as one serving?

Breads, Cereals, Rice and Pasta
– 1 slice of bread
– ½ cup of cooked rice or pasta
– ½ cup of cooked cereal
– 1 ounce of ready-to-eat cereal

Fruits
– 1 piece of fruit or melon wedge
– ¾ cup of juice
– ½ cup of canned fruit
– ½ cup of dried fruit

Fats, Oils and Sweets
– Limit calories from these, especially if you need to lose weight

Vegetables
– ½ cup of chopped raw or cooked vegetables
– 1 cup of leafy raw vegetables

Milk, Yogurt and Cheese
– 1 cup of milk or yogurt
– 1½ to 2 ounces of cheese

Meat, Poultry, Fish, Dry Beans, Eggs and Nuts
– 2½ to 3 ounces of cooked lean meat, poultry or fish
– Count ½ cup of cooked beans or 1 egg, or 2 table spoons of peanut butter as 1 ounce of lean meat (about a third of a serving)

The amount you eat may be more than one serving, for example , a dinner portion of spaghetti would count as two or three servings of pasta.

A Closer Look at Fat and Added Sugars

The small tip of the Food Guide Pyramid shows fats, oils and sweets. These are foods such as salad dressings, cream, butter, margarine, sugars, soft drinks, candies and sweet desserts. Alcoholic beverages are also part of this group. These foods provide calories but few vitamins and minerals. Most people should go easy on foods from this group.

Some fat or sugar symbols are show in other food groups. That's to remind you that some foods in these groups can also be high in fat and added sugars, such as cheese or ice cream from the milk group or french fries from the vegetable group. When choosing foods for a healthful diet, consider the fat and added sugars in your choices from all the food groups, not just fats, oils and sweets.

Appendix G: Body-Mass Index

Age	19	20	21	22	23	24	25	26	27	28	29	30	35	40
Height (inches)							Weight (pounds)							
58	91	95	100	105	110	115	119	124	129	134	138	143	167	191
59	94	99	104	109	114	119	124	128	133	138	143	148	173	196
60	97	102	107	112	118	123	128	133	138	143	148	153	179	204
61	100	106	111	116	121	127	132	137	143	148	153	158	185	211
62	104	113	115	120	125	131	136	142	147	153	158	164	191	218
63	107	109	118	124	130	135	141	146	152	158	163	169	197	225
64	110	116	122	128	134	140	145	151	157	163	169	174	203	233
65	114	120	126	132	138	144	150	156	162	168	174	180	210	240
66	117	124	130	136	142	148	155	161	167	173	179	185	216	247
67	121	127	134	140	147	153	159	166	172	178	185	191	223	255
68	125	131	138	144	151	158	164	171	177	184	190	197	230	263
69	128	135	142	149	155	162	169	176	182	189	196	203	237	270
70	132	139	146	153	160	167	174	181	188	195	202	209	243	278
71	136	143	150	157	165	172	179	186	193	200	207	215	250	286
72	140	147	155	162	169	177	184	191	199	206	213	221	258	294
73	144	151	159	166	174	182	189	197	204	212	219	227	265	303
74	148	155	163	171	179	187	194	202	210	218	225	233	272	311
75	152	160	168	176	184	192	200	208	216	224	232	240	279	319
76	156	164	172	180	189	197	205	213	221	230	238	246	287	328

NOTE: *Suppose your height is 70" and you weigh 174 pounds. To determine your Body-Mass Index (BMI) from this chart, find your height (70") in the far left column. Read across that row in the chart until you find your weight (174). Then, read up that column to the top to find your BMI (25).*

Appendix H: Vitamin Facts

VITAMIN	U.S. RDA*	BEST SOURCES	FUNCTIONS
A (carotene)	5,000 IU/day	Yellow or orange fruits and vegetables, green leafy vegetables, fortified oatmeal, liver, daily products	Formation and maintance of skin, hair and mucous membranes; helps vision in dim light; bone and tooth growth
B1 (thiamine)	1.2 mg/day	Fortified cereals and oatmeals, meats, rice and pasta, whole grains, liver	Helps body release energy from carbohydrates during metabolism; growth and muscle tone
B2 (riboflavin)	1.3 mg/day	Whole grains, green leafy vegetables, organ meats, milk and eggs	Helps body release energy from protein, fat and carbohydrates during metabolism
B6 (pyridoxine)	1.3 mg/day	Fish, poultry, lean meats, bananas, prunes, dried beans, whole grains, avocados	Helps build body tissue and aids in metabolism of protein
B12 (cobalamin)	2.4 mcg/day	Meats, milk products, seafood	Aids cell development, functioning of the nervous system and the metabolism of protein and fat
Biotin	30 mcg/day	Cereal/grain products, seafood	Involved in metabolism of protein, fats and carbohydrates
Folate (folacin, folic acid)	400 mcg/day	Green leafy vegetables, organ meats, dried peas, beans and lentils	Aids in genetic material development; involved in red blood cell production
Niacin	16 mg/day	Meat, poultry, fish, enriched cereals, peanuts, potatoes, dairy products, eggs	Involved in carbohydrate, protein and fat metabolism
Pantothenic Acid	5 mg/day	Lean meats, whole grains, legumes, vegetables, fruits	Helps in the release of energy from fats and carboydrates
C (ascorbic acid)	90 mg/day	Citrus fruits, berries and vegetables—especially peppers	Essential for structure of bones, cartilage, muscle and blood vessels; helps maintain capillaries and gums; aids in absorption of iron

Vitamin Facts (continued)

VITAMIN	U.S. RDA*	BEST SOURCES	FUNCTIONS
D	400 IU/day	Fortified milk, sunlight, fish, eggs, butter, fortified margarine	Aids in bone and tooth formation; helps maintain heart action and nervous system
E	30 IU/day	Fortified and multi-grain cereals, nuts, wheat germ, vegetable oils, green leafy vegetables	Protects blood cells, body tissue and essential fatty acids from harmful destruction in the body
K	**	Green leafy vegetables, fruit, dairy and grain products	Essential for blood clotting functions

For adults and children over 19. IU= international units; mg=milligrams; mcg= micrograms

Mineral Facts

MINERAL	U.S. RDA*	BEST SOURCES	FUNCTIONS
Calcium	1000 mg/day	Milk and milk products	Strong bones, teeth, muscle tissue; regulates heart beat, muscle action and nerve function; blood clotting
Chromium	35 mcg/day	Corn oil, clams, whole grain cereals, brewer's yeast	Glucose metabolism (energy); increases effectiveness of insulin
Copper	900 mcg/day	Oysters, nuts, organ meats, legumes	Formation of red blood cells, bone growth and health; works with vitamin C to form elastin
Iodine	150 mcg/day	Seafood, iodized salt	Strong bones, teeth and muscle tissue; regulates heart beat, muscle action and nerve function; blood clotting
Iron	18 mg/day	Meats and organ meats, legumes	Hemoglobin formation; improves blood quality; increases resistance to stress and disease

BE FIT, STAY FIT!

Mineral Facts (continued)

MINERAL	U.S. RDA*	BEST SOURCES	FUNCTIONS
Magnesuim	400 mg/day	Nuts, green vegetables, whole grains	Acid/alkaline balance; important in metabolism of carbohydrates, minerals and sugar
Manganese	2.3 mg/day	Nuts, whole grains, vegetables, fruits	Enzyme activation; carbohydrate and fat production; sex hormone production; skeletal development
Phosphorus	700 mg/day	Fish, meat, poultry, eggs, grains	Bone development; important in protein, fat and carbohydrate utilization
Potassium	No RDA	Lean meat, vegetables, fruits	Fluid balance; controls activity of heart muscle, nervous system and kidneys
Selenium	55 mcg/day	Seafood, organ meats, lean meats, grains	Protects body tissues against oxidative domage from radiation and pollution aids in normal metabolic processing
Zinc	11 mg/day	Lean meats, liver, eggs, seafood, whole grains	Involved in digestion and metaboilsm; important in development of reproductive system; aids in healing

Source: The American Institute of Cancer Research

Appendix I: The Fitness Points Log

FITNESS ACTIVITY	SUNDAY	MONDAY	TUESDAY	WEDNESDAY	THURSDAY	FRIDAY	SATURDAY	WEEKLY TOTAL
Strength Training (with proper form)								
Cardiovascular Training								
Flexibility/Stretching								
Diet/Eating Plan								
Other								
Weekly Grand Total								

The Fitness Points Log Scoring System

Strength Training (with proper form)
1 point per body part per day
    Maximum: 6 points per day/24 points per week

Cardiovascular Training
1 point per every 10 minutes each day (brisk walking, running, hiking, swimming, stepping machines, group fitness classes, etc.)
    Maximum: 6 points per day/30 points per week
    Example: 1 hour group fitness class – 6 points
                30 minutes treadmill at target heart rate – 3 points

Flexibility/Stretching
1 point per every 15 minutes stretching/flexibility exercise
    Maximum: 4 points per day/20 points per week
    Example: 1 hour yoga class – 4 points
                15 minutes stretching after workout – 1 point

Diet/Eating Plan
1 point for each day not exceeding suggested calorie level (See Food Pyramid Guide for details)
1 point for each of six groups checked off as adequate on the Eating Plan Analysis (see Appendix E).

Appendix I: The Fitness Points Log (cont.)

Maximum: 7 points per day/49 points per week

Other
1 point for each of the following:
- Gardening/yard work per hour
- Mowing the lawn (non-riding mower) per hour
- Taking the stairs (minimum 3 flights per day)
- Housework (active involvement) per hour
- Walking 1000 steps (at work, at home or at the mall, etc.) *Note: 1000 steps is equivalent to one-third or one-half of a mile depending on stride length.*
- Calisthenic Exercise per 15 minutes

Maximum: 6 points per day

Weekly Fitness Points Program Ratings
  120 and Higher: Superior
  100 to 119: Great
  80-99: Good
  60-79: Room for Improvement
  40-59: Borderline "Couch Potato"
  20-39: Poor
  Less than 20: Dangerous

The Fitness Points Log can be downloaded at www.cardinalpub.com/befit

Appendix J: Workout Card

BODY PART: Exercise/Lift	Month /Day					
CHEST: (2)						
* Chest Press/Bench Press 8-12 repetitions BB, M, DB						
Bent Arm Press 8-12 repetitions BB, M						
UPPER BACK: (2)						
Lat Pulldown 8-12 repetitions M						
* Seated Row 8-12 repetitions M						
Bent Over Row 8-12 repetitions DB						
Pullover 8-12 repetitions M						
SHOULDERS:						
Lateral Raise 8-12 repetitions DB, M						
* Seated Press 8-12 repetitions DB, BB, M						
Upright Row 8-12 repetitions BB						
HIPS:						
Squat 10-15, 15-20 repetitions BB						
* Leg Press 10-15, 15-20 repetitions M						
LEGS:						
* Leg Extension 10-15 repetitions M						
* Leg Curl 10-15 repetitions M						

Appendix J: Workout Card (cont.)

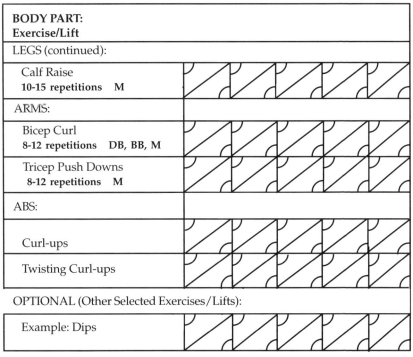

BODY PART: Exercise/Lift						
LEGS (continued):						
Calf Raise **10-15 repetitions M**						
ARMS:						
Bicep Curl **8-12 repetitions DB, BB, M**						
Tricep Push Downs **8-12 repetitions M**						
ABS:						
Curl-ups						
Twisting Curl-ups						
OPTIONAL (Other Selected Exercises/Lifts):						
Example: Dips						

Modality Codes: BB= barbell, DB= dumbell, M= selectorized machine, Reps 8-12, 10-15, 15-20. Remember reminder to use the proper technique and to warm up and cool down before and after working out. The * designates items that are part of the core workout. **A full page (8½ x 11) copy of this chart is available at www.cardinalpub.com/befit.**

Sample

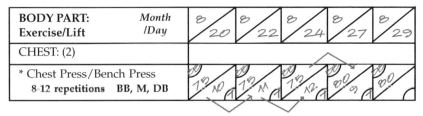

BODY PART: Exercise/Lift	Month /Day	8 20	8 22	8 24	8 27	8 29
CHEST: (2)						
* Chest Press/Bench Press **8-12 repetitions BB, M, DB**						

Figure 3.5: Workout Card with Sample Data. Notice the increase in weight or resistance and the increase in repetitions. On 8/29, note that the resistance is already recorded for the next workout.